JOSLIN'S GUIDE TO

Managing Childhood Diabetes

A Family Teamwork Approach

Lori M. B. Laffel, MD, MPH
Deborah A. Butler, MSW, LICSW, CDE
Laurie A. Higgins, MS, RD, LDN, CDE
Margaret T. Lawlor, MS, CDE
Cynthia A. Pasquarello, BSN, RN, CDE

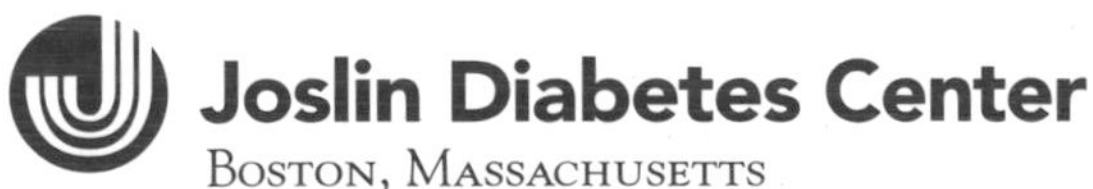

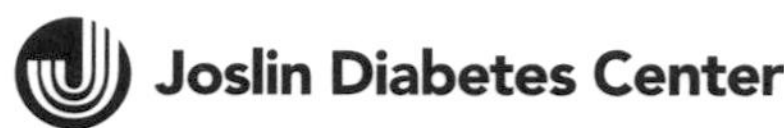

Published by Joslin Diabetes Center, Boston, MA
Web site: www.joslin.org

ISBN: 978-1-879091-37-5

Joslin Diabetes Center
Publications Department
One Joslin Place
Boston, MA 02215

The publisher offers discounts on this book when ordered in bulk quantities.
For information, contact the Joslin Publications Department at the address above or call 617-226-5815.

TABLE OF CONTENTS

Letter from Dr. Laffel

Dear Parents, Families of Children with Diabetes, School Personnel and Educators,

Welcome! We created *Joslin's Guide to Managing Childhood Diabetes – A Family Teamwork Approach* to provide you with the most current information about caring for children, adolescents and young adults with diabetes. In this book, you will find strategies, tips and tools – all to help the child in your care achieve the mutual goals of maintaining normal growth and development, successful schooling, outstanding physical fitness, and just having fun being a child or teen.

Joslin's Guide to Managing Childhood Diabetes – A Family Teamwork Approach was developed with the support of the Kevin Youkilis Hits for Kids Foundation because Kevin and his team are dedicated to helping children and teens be the best that they can be at managing their diabetes.

Diabetes is not a do-it-yourself condition at any age, but especially not for children. Children and teens need support for successful diabetes management. We at Joslin Pediatrics wanted to create a book that draws on our experience and gives you the tools to deliver that support. Our recommendations will help your family, school and community work together with your healthcare team to make diabetes fit into your life, rather than make your life fit into the diabetes treatment plan.

In this book, you will learn what diabetes is and how to treat it. You will learn about various insulins; the different ways to deliver insulin, whether by syringe, pen or pump; and approaches to healthy eating and physical activity. Some sections of the book focus on care, other sections review diabetes cure and prevention research, and others discuss ways to support the child or teen with diabetes at home with the family, at school, and in the community. You will learn about approaches to checking glucose levels, new medications, and how to advise children to keep their bodies healthy.

It is with ongoing education and support that children will succeed in school and continue on a path for a successful future. Children with diabetes and their families need extra education and support to find the best approach to diabetes management. I encourage you to use the book as a management tool and as a reference when questions arise. Share various chapters with your school, your child's coach, or other members of the community as you see fit.

The members of the Joslin Diabetes Center Pediatric Team express our deepest thanks to Kevin Youkilis and the Hits for Kids Foundation for providing us with the resources to write and publish this book.

Sincerely,

Lori Laffel

Lori Laffel, M.D., M.P.H.
Chief, Pediatric and Adolescent and Young Adult Section
Joslin Diabetes Center

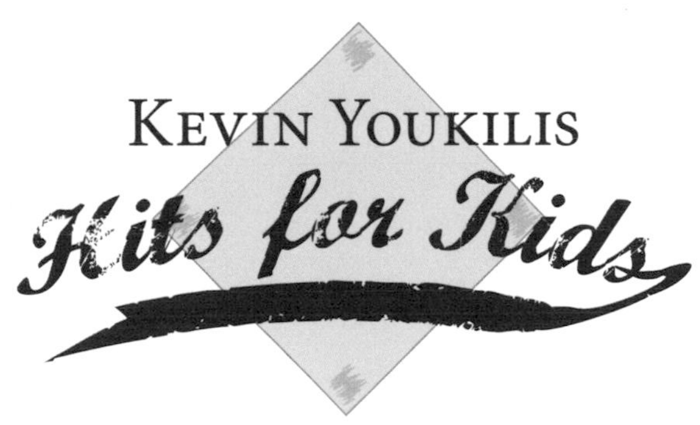

Founded by Boston Red Sox first baseman Kevin Youkilis and his wife, Enza, Kevin Youkilis *Hits for Kids* is a non-profit organization that works to garner individual and corporate support for local charities and organizations that work to improve the health and well-being of children. Youk's Kids partners with existing community-based children's charities and medical research programs in New England to help them raise money and awareness. Through our careful selection process, we have been able to impact the lives of so many children who rarely get the support they desperately need. These organizations include Christopher's Haven, Italian Home for Children, Nativity Preparatory School, Birthday Wishes, Lovelane, and, of course, Joslin Diabetes Center's Pediatric Health Services.

Youk's Kids has had the honor of partnering with Joslin since its inception, in part because Kevin and his family have been personally affected by diabetes; and also because of the growing incidence of diabetes among children in America. As we continue our mission to help children in need, we remain dedicated to supporting Joslin so it can offer kids with diabetes the support and knowledge they need to cope with their disease.

To learn more about Kevin Youkilis *Hits for Kids*, please visit: www.youkskids.org or call 617.444.9685.

Letter from Kevin Youkilis

To those who care for children with diabetes,

As adults, we are in the position to foster safe, nurturing and healthy environments for children. That's the principal behind the Kevin Youkilis Hits for Kids foundation, and that is why we support the Joslin Diabetes Center's Pediatric Health Services.

When Dr. Lori Laffel told us of the increasing incidence of diabetes among children, we knew we needed to get involved. And when she told us that *Joslin's Guide to Managing Childhood Diabetes* would help adults better care for children with diabetes, we knew it would be a home run and wanted to get behind it.

As you read this manual and discuss elements of it with your kids, please tell them that while I don't have diabetes, I care for my body by eating right and getting plenty of exercise so that when I walk out onto the field with the Boston Red Sox, I can do my best.

Just like Dr. Lori Laffel and the Pediatrics team at Joslin, the Kevin Youkilis Hits for Kids Foundation goes to bat every day for kids with diabetes.

Sincerely,
Kevin Youkilis

CONTRIBUTING AUTHORS

Kristen N. Bruneau, BA, CCLS
Child Life Specialist, Care Ambassador
Joslin Diabetes Center

Deborah A. Butler, MSW, LICSW, CDE
Associate Director, Pediatric Programs
Joslin Diabetes Center
Instructor in Psychiatry
Harvard Medical School

Jennifer Douglass, MEd, CCLS
Child Life Specialist, Care Ambassador
Joslin Diabetes Center

Elizabeth Foster, BSN, RN
Pediatric and Adolescent Nurse Specialist
Joslin Diabetes Center

Laurie A. Higgins, MS, RD, LDN, CDE
Pediatric Nutrition & Diabetes Educator
Joslin Diabetes Center

Deborah Lees Holtorf, MPH, MSN, PNP-BC, BC-ADM
Pediatric and Adolescent Nurse Specialist
Joslin Diabetes Center

Kendra Juhola Magyar, RN, MSN, PNP-BC
Pediatric and Adolescent Nurse Specialist
Research Nurse
Joslin Diabetes Center

Joyce Keady, RN, MSN, CPNP
Pediatric and Adolescent Nurse Specialist
Research Nurse
Joslin Diabetes Center

Lisa Kuhn, BSN, RN
Pediatric and Adolescent Nurse Specialist
Research Nurse
Joslin Diabetes Center

Lori M. B. Laffel, MD, MPH
Chief, Pediatric, Adolescent, and Young Adult Section
Joslin Diabetes Center
Associate Professor of Pediatrics
Harvard Medical School

Margaret T. Lawlor, MS, CDE
Coordinator of Pediatric Research & Education
Joslin Diabetes Center

M. Joan Mansfield, MD
Associate Clinical Director of Pediatrics
Joslin Diabetes Center
Assistant Professor of Pediatrics
Harvard Medical School

Sanjeev N. Mehta, MD, MPH
Research Associate and Staff Physician
Joslin Diabetes Center
Instructor in Pediatrics
Harvard Medical School

Kerry Milaszewski, BS, RN, CDE
Pediatric and Adolescent Nurse Specialist
Research Nurse
Joslin Diabetes Center

Cynthia A. Pasquarello, BSN, RN, CDE
Nurse Manager, Pediatric, Adolescent, and Young Adult Section
Joslin Diabetes Center

Amy Pettit, PhD
Psychology Fellow
Joslin Diabetes Center

Alyne T. Ricker, MD
Staff Physician
Joslin Diabetes Center
Instructor in Pediatrics
Harvard Medical School

Britta Svoren, MD
Staff Physician
Joslin Diabetes Center
Instructor in Pediatrics
Harvard Medical School

Christina Von Seggern, MSN, APRN, FNP-BC
Pediatric and Adolescent Nurse Specialist
Research Nurse
Joslin Diabetes Center

Emily Werner, MS, RD, LDN, CDE
Pediatric Nutrition & Diabetes Educator
Joslin Diabetes Center

JOSLIN'S GUIDE TO

Managing Childhood Diabetes

1

Diabetes — What is it?

Childhood diabetes is a long-term chronic disorder that results from the body's inability to use sugar for energy. Sugar, known as glucose (and glucose will be the term used throughout this book) is derived from carbohydrates in the foods we eat. In order to use energy from carbohydrates, the hormone insulin is needed to allow the glucose molecules to enter the body's cells. The cells then use the glucose to release energy for the body's ongoing processes of growth, repair, and maintenance. When one has diabetes, inadequate insulin production by the pancreas or inadequate insulin usage by the body causes the blood glucose to rise to an unhealthy level. Diabetes can develop at any age. This book focuses on type 1 diabetes in the child, adolescent, and young-adult. Please note as you read this book that we recognize and celebrate the diverse make-up of families who are affected by diabetes. But to simplify writing, when we refer to parent and child in the following pages, we are referring to all primary caretakers and the many ages and stages, from birth to young adulthood.

There is no cure for diabetes. However, we have outstanding treatment tools that allow children with diabetes to maintain normal growth and development, to participate fully in school and athletic activities, and to mature into young, productive, and healthy adults. Though children with diabetes are faced with the usual psychosocial and behavioral trials and tribulations of each developmental stage, living with diabetes does provide unique challenges along the way. To help overcome these challenges, diverse diabetes management strategies are used, which are directed to the individual needs of the child and family as they progress through development. We emphasize the importance of the family's management of diabetes and its evolution into diabetes self-management, taking into account that diabetes is not a do-it-yourself condition at any age. It truly takes a village to raise a child with diabetes, as the day-to-day rigors of diabetes management are best met with a team approach to care and ongoing family support. With such an approach, the gifts of long-term health and well-being are possible with today's diabetes treatment tools.

What is Diabetes?

The purpose of this chapter is to provide answers to some of the questions that parents commonly ask after being told that their child has diabetes. Let's start with some basics.

1. **What is diabetes?** Diabetes mellitus is a chronic condition characterized by elevated levels of glucose (sugar) in the blood. Diabetes requires life-long therapy.
2. **How is diabetes diagnosed?** Diabetes is diagnosed in 1 of 4 ways. All 4 ways are based on the level of glucose in the blood.
   a. Method One: A child exhibits what are considered the classic symptoms of diabetes (*e.g.*, increased thirst, increased urination, unexplained weight loss) and has a random blood glucose level greater than or equal to 200 mg/dL. (Confirmed in a laboratory, not by home blood glucose meter.)
   b. Method Two: When a child has not had anything to eat or drink for at least 8 hours and a fasting glucose reading obtained after that 8-hour period is greater than or equal to 126 mg/dL.
   c. Method Three: The results of a specialized test called an oral glucose tolerance test indicate diabetes. During this test, after an 8-hour fast, a child is asked to drink a sugary drink of glucose dissolved in water. Diabetes is diagnosed if the child's blood glucose level is greater than or equal to 200 mg/dL 2 hours after the solution is consumed.
   d. Method Four: A laboratory drawn A1C (times 2) is greater than or equal to 6.5%.

If there is any question about the diagnosis, your child's medical provider might suggest ordering more tests or repeating the same tests on a different day to see if similar results are achieved.

3. **What is insulin?** In order to understand what causes the blood glucose levels to rise in a child with diabetes, you need to learn about insulin and the important role that it plays in the body.
   a. Insulin is a hormone that is made and released by the beta cells of the pancreas.
   b. The main function of insulin is to lower the level of glucose in the blood as it starts to rise.
   c. In addition, insulin turns off the body's production of glucose from the breakdown of fuel stored in tissues such as liver, muscle, and fat.
   d. After a person eats a meal and digestion begins, glucose is absorbed into the blood. If a person has not recently eaten, the liver starts to release its stores of glucose into the blood.
   e. Regardless of the source of the glucose, the job of insulin is to transport the glucose out of the blood and into the cells of the body where it can be used for energy.
   f. In other words, insulin is the key that unlocks the door to the cell and allows glucose to enter and provide it with energy.
   g. Without insulin, the door to the cell stays locked and glucose is unable to leave the blood.
4. **Are there different types of diabetes?** There are different types of diabetes that can affect children. Typically, diabetes is classified as type 1, type 2, or other specific types.
   a. *Type 1 diabetes*. This condition is caused by the destruction of pancreatic beta cells by the body's immune system. Unfortunately, nobody understands exactly why this occurs. Both genetic and environmental factors are thought to be involved. Although the rest of the pancreas continues to work normally, the beta cells are destroyed and lose their ability to make insulin. Therefore, insulin levels in the body are very low. Until recently, almost all children diagnosed with diabetes had type 1 diabetes.
   b. *Type 2 diabetes*. Over the past 10-20 years, more children in the United States and elsewhere in the world have been diagnosed with type 2 diabetes. In children with this condition, the beta cells are not destroyed by the immune system. The beta cells

continue to make insulin; however, the body is resistant to the effects of the insulin. In other words, the body is unable to use the insulin properly. Unlike children with type 1 diabetes, children with type 2 diabetes usually have normal or elevated serum insulin levels because the body is working hard to try and overcome its resistance to the insulin. The worldwide problem of overweight and obesity is largely responsible for the increasing number of children and adolescents who are developing type 2 diabetes.

   c. Other specific types. All other known causes of diabetes fall into this third category.
      i. *Maturity Onset Diabetes of the Young* (MODY) is an inherited genetic disorder of beta cells. In this condition, the beta cell is not destroyed, but it is unable to function properly to make or release insulin.
      ii. Diabetes that develops following *surgical removal of the pancreas* is another example of a condition that would fall into this category.
      iii. *Neonatal Diabetes* is diagnosed shortly after birth and almost always within the first six months of life. This unique type of diabetes results from a genetic defect that prevents the insulin producing beta cells from releasing insulin. While infants diagnosed with diabetes will need insulin initially, once the infant/child is stabilized and the diagnosis of neonatal diabetes is confirmed, the insulin can often be replaced by a pill to maintain blood glucose levels. The diagnosis of this rare condition is confirmed by special genetic testing.

5. **What are the stages of type 1 diabetes?** The 4 stages of diabetes are:
   a. *Onset* – Symptoms such as increased thirst, increased urination, weight loss or poor weight gain, etc., tell you that something is not right with your child.
   b. *Honeymoon* – Once a child starts on insulin shots, the remaining beta cells get a rest and allow the pancreas to produce some insulin for a time.
   c. *Intensification* – Insulin producing beta cell destruction contin-

ues. It becomes more difficult to keep the child's blood glucose in range.

d. *Total Diabetes* – All or most of the insulin producing beta cells in the pancreas have been destroyed. Insulin needs increase with growth.

6. **How do I know what type of diabetes my child has?** Your child's medical provider is likely to take a number of factors into consideration when determining what type of diabetes your child has. These factors include details about your child's medical history, physical examination, and laboratory studies.

7. **What are some of the most important factors that are likely to be taken into consideration?**

   a. *Body type*. Children with type 1 diabetes are not usually overweight and often have a recent history of weight loss. In comparison, children with type 2 diabetes are generally overweight. It is important to understand, however, that a child can be overweight and still be diagnosed with type 1 diabetes.

   b. *Age*. Although a child is most likely to be diagnosed with type 1 diabetes during 2 periods in his or her life — between the ages of 4 and 6-years old, and then between 10 and 14-years old when most children start to enter or are in the early stages of puberty — a diagnosis of diabetes can occur at any age. In comparison, children with type 2 diabetes are usually diagnosed after the onset of puberty. It would be unusual for a young child who has not yet entered puberty to be diagnosed with type 2 diabetes. However, it is important to keep in mind that there is significant overlap between the two types of diabetes.

   c. *Ethnicity*. In the United States, most children diagnosed with type 1 diabetes are Caucasian. In comparison, most children diagnosed with type 2 diabetes belong to minority ethnic groups, including African Americans, Hispanics, Native Americans, and Asian Americans. Once again, however, there is significant overlap between the two types of diabetes.

   d. *Insulin resistance*. Upon physical examination, children with type 2 diabetes usually have signs that suggest they have insulin resistance. For example, sometimes there is a darkening and/or a thickening of the skin (called *acanthosis nigricans*) on the back of the neck or under the arms that suggests insulin resistance. This condition is not commonly seen in children with type 1 diabetes.

e. *Auto-antibodies*. Type 1 diabetes is suggested by the detection of pancreatic auto-antibodies in the blood. After cells from the body's immune system damage the beta cells, different cells from the immune system make antibodies. The names of these antibodies include anti-insulin antibody, GAD antibody, and IA2 antibody. More than 80% of children with type 1 diabetes will have 1 or more of these antibodies in their blood. With newer antibodies (zinc channel) available in research laboratories, more than 90% of youth with diabetes will have detectable auto-antibodies. The presence of serum auto-antibodies makes the diagnosis of other types of diabetes less likely.

f. *Other useful blood tests*. The level of insulin in the blood, if obtained before a child is started on insulin injections, can sometimes be useful in distinguishing between type 1 and type 2 diabetes. In children with type 1 diabetes, the insulin level is usually low or undetectable. In children with type 2 diabetes, the insulin level is usually normal or elevated. Sometimes the level of C-peptide level in the child's blood can also be useful in distinguishing between the different types of diabetes. C-peptide is part of the natural insulin molecule produced by the beta cell but is not part of the synthetic insulin molecule that is given by injection. Similar to insulin, C-peptide levels are usually low or undetectable in children with type 1 diabetes and normal or elevated in children with type 2 diabetes. This test is especially useful in the child who has been started on insulin injections.

g. *Genetic tests*. If your child's medical provider has reason to suspect that your child has one of the rarer forms of diabetes (*e.g.*, MODY, neo-natal diabetes), he or she may suggest obtaining certain genetic tests. These tests examine your child's DNA for potential defects that do not allow your child's beta cells to function properly to make or release insulin.

8. **What are the symptoms of diabetes?** Regardless of the type of diabetes, the symptoms that a child may experience are usually quite similar. If a child's pancreas is unable to make insulin (type 1 diabetes), or if a child's body is unable to use insulin properly (type 2 diabetes), glucose builds up in the blood.
   a. Once the amount of glucose in the blood rises above a certain level, the body begins to rid itself of the excess amount by passing it out through urine. More frequent urination is the result.
   b. Increased thirst, which is the body's way of protecting against dehydration, develops in response to the increased urination and prompts a person to drink more fluids. This explains why two of the most common symptoms a parent will notice are that the child who is developing diabetes is drinking and urinating more than usual.
   c. At the same time that these processes are occurring, the body's cells begin to get hungry because they are not receiving glucose and they need to turn to other sources of stored energy, primarily in the form of fat, for food. As fat gets broken down, ketones are produced, and the child commonly begins to lose weight. The child may also complain of feeling more tired than usual. If the ketones in the blood reach a high level, abdominal pain, nausea, and vomiting can result. The child's breath may also take on a sweet smell. Ketones tend to form more easily in the child who is unable to make insulin than in the child who is resistant to the action of insulin. The only way to stop ketones from being produced is to replace the insulin that the body is missing. After a child is diagnosed with diabetes and insulin treatment is begun, ketones gradually disappear, blood glucose values decrease, increased thirst and urination return to normal, and weight is gained back.

Table 1-1. Symptoms of Diabetes

Thirst	Hunger (sometimes no hunger at all)
Increased urination (trouble toilet training or bedwetting)	Weight loss or poor weight gain
Blurred vision	Nausea and/or vomiting
Mood swings	

9. **How is diabetes treated?** The type of diabetes a child has often determines what type of treatment works best. Although the treatment of diabetes will be discussed in much greater detail in the chapters that follow, a brief overview is provided here.
   a. *Type 1 diabetes*. Because the pancreas of a child with type 1 diabetes is no longer able to make enough insulin to keep the blood glucose levels in range, he or she needs to be started on insulin therapy. No other options exist. Insulin has been available since 1922, and major advances in its use have been made over the past 20 years. Insulin can only be given by injection. You can't give insulin as a pill because the acid in the stomach would destroy it. The aim of insulin therapy in the treatment of diabetes is to mimic the changes in insulin levels in the blood that are seen in individuals who do not have diabetes. In order to do so, most children with type 1 diabetes either need to receive three or more injections of insulin each day or use an insulin pump, a mechanical device the size of a small mobile phone worn by the child at all times. Your child's medical provider will help you to determine what type of insulin regimen is likely to be best for your child and your lifestyle.
   b. *Type 2 diabetes*. Because the pancreas of a child with type 2 diabetes is still able to produce insulin, insulin replacement therapy is often not needed. Instead, the child can be treated with a pill or liquid that is taken by mouth and helps the body to use its own insulin more effectively.
   c. If it is unclear whether a child has type 1 or type 2 diabetes, he or she is usually started on insulin but then switched to an oral medication once the diagnosis of type 2 diabetes is confirmed. However, the opposite can also happen. A child with type 2 diabetes might be started on an oral medication, but insulin might be added later if the medication is unable to adequately control the blood glucose levels. Also, children with type 2 diabetes often receive insulin therapy initially, which can later be weaned after blood glucose levels are controlled.

10. **Who develops diabetes?** You might be surprised to learn that diabetes is one of the most common chronic diseases affecting children and adolescents today.
    a. According to recent data, approximately 1 out of every 300 youth in the United States age 10-19 years has diabetes. The SEARCH for Diabetes in Youth Study estimated that in 2001 there were close to 200,000 children and adolescents with diabetes living in the United States.
    b. You also might also be interested to learn that the incidence of childhood type 1 diabetes has increased worldwide over the last half-century. In particular, there has been a sharp rise in the number of children under 6 years of age who have been developing type 1 diabetes over the last 2 decades. Unfortunately we do not know why this is occurring. Various environmental factors (e.g., infections, toxins, foods, cow's milk, immunizations, stress) have been explored, however we still do not have the answer.

It is important to know that nothing you did as parents caused your child to develop type 1 diabetes. Nor was there anything you could have done to prevent your child from developing type 1 diabetes.

As mentioned previously, the increased occurrence of type 2 diabetes in children and adolescents follows the epidemic of childhood overweight and obesity. Over the past 2 decades, the number of children in the United States who are overweight or obese has doubled. Currently, 1 out of every 3 children is either overweight or obese. Before the 1990s, it was rare for most pediatric diabetes centers to have patients with type 2 diabetes. By 1994, type 2 diabetes accounted for up to 16% of all new cases of diabetes in children living in urban areas. In order to address the problem of type 2 diabetes in children and adolescents, we need to address the underlying problem of childhood obesity.

Summary

Unfortunately, at the present time, there is no cure for diabetes. However, there are currently many researchers, working at Joslin Diabetes Center and elsewhere around the world, who are trying to better understand what causes diabetes. The hope is that if scientists can better understand what causes diabetes, they might be able to develop ways to either prevent or cure it.

References and Resources

Dabelea D, Bell RA, D'Agostino RB, Jr., Imperatore G, Johansen JM, Linder B et al. Incidence of diabetes in youth in the United States. *JAMA*. 2007;297(24):2716-2724.

Liese AD, D'Agostino RB, Jr., Hamman RF, Kilgo PD, Lawrence JM, Liu LL et al. The burden of diabetes mellitus among US youth: prevalence estimates from the SEARCH for Diabetes in Youth Study. *Pediatrics*. 2006;118(4):1510-1518.

Gale EA. The rise of childhood type 1 diabetes in the 20th century. *Diabetes*. 2002;51(12):3353-3361.

EURODIAB ACE study group. Variation and trends in incidence of childhood diabetes in Europe. EURODIAB ACE Study Group. *Lancet*. 2000;355(9207):873-876.

Rosenbloom A.L., Joe J.R., Young R.S., Winter W.E. Emerging epidemic of type 2 diabetes in youth. *Diabetes Care*. 1999;22(2):345-354.

Daniels SR, Greer FR. Lipid screening and cardiovascular health in childhood. *Pediatrics*. 2008;122(1):198-208.

Web sites:

- Joslin Diabetes Center: www.joslin.org
- American Diabetes Association: www.diabetes.org
- Children with Diabetes: www.childrenwithdiabetes.com

2

The Team Approach and Tools of Diabetes Management

Managing diabetes is complex. You need to know how to check blood glucose, draw up insulin, give your child injections, figure out what a carbohydrate is, identify a carbohydrate from a protein, recognize your child's symptoms of a low blood glucose and how to treat it . . . and the list goes on. With all this information, families with diabetes must figure out how they are going to learn to keep up with all things diabetes and still manage the rest of life in general — and your child's life in particular.

Take a moment to take several deep breaths and exhale slowly. You and your child are not alone! No one expects that you will learn everything in a week or even in a month. Diabetes education starts with survival education and continues with ongoing education as your child evolves throughout the normal cycles of childhood, adolescence, and early adulthood. Being a parent does not mean that you know everything — your kids will remind you of that fact anyway.

Caring for Your Child's Diabetes

The African proverb "It takes an entire village to raise a single child" rings true in diabetes care; it takes an entire diabetes healthcare team to care for and empower a child with diabetes and his or her family. You are going to meet a whole team of people who are here to support you and your child as you learn about diabetes.

The Team Approach

Since diabetes affects all aspects of your child's life, the support of family and guidance of the healthcare team is required for a successful outcome. The team approach is particularly critical in the current era of intensive insulin therapy, in which insulin is administered frequently in an effort to match the body's usual insulin production. Intensive insulin therapy requires complex medical management, including frequent blood glucose monitoring, timely administration of insulin, provision of regular meals and snacks with known carbohydrate amounts, and an exercise program that becomes as much therapeutic as recreational in nature.

Strategies for managing diabetes change as your child grows and develops, as do the feelings you and your child have about living with diabetes. The variety of skills provided by a multidisciplinary team is called into play as these changes occur. You and your child are the most important members of this team. To provide high-quality diabetes education, educational goals should be established by members of the diabetes care team through meetings with both the child and his or her family. Depending on the child's age at diagnosis, he or she will be asked to participate in his or her care, because to be effective, medical care and diabetes education that is geared toward the family must appropriately include the child.

Diabetes treatment and self-management education will generally take place during clinic visits. During such visits, a variety of multidisciplinary healthcare team members may be seen. Your pediatric endocrinologist and pediatric diabetes nurse educator will help you and your child recognize when you need the services of each of these team members as well as other specialists identified later. Your primary healthcare team members include:

- Physicians/Doctors
- Nurses/Nurse Practitioners
- Dietitians
- Psychologists and Social Workers
- Child Life Specialists

- Medical Assistants
- Pediatric Phlebotomists
- Exercise Physiologists
- Office staff

Your child's team also includes other people who interact with him or her on a frequent basis and can help support the child as needed. These medical and non-medical team members include:

- Family — notably parents, grandparents, aunts, uncles, siblings, and family friends
- Members of the school staff including:
  - School Nurses
  - Teachers
  - Coaches
  - Secretaries
  - Cafeteria Staff
  - Bus Drivers
  - Others

The primary multidisciplinary team named above has expertise in multiple aspects of pediatric diabetes management, but as your child grows and has lived longer with diabetes, there are other medical specialists who may be called upon to assist in your child's care. They include:

- Ophthalmologists/Optometrist
- Podiatrists
- Nephrologists
- Neurologists
- Gastroenterologists

Your healthcare team is responsible for helping your family make its way through the healthcare system. The following describes in greater detail the roles of some of the primary team members you will encounter as you continue your journey with diabetes:

- **Pediatric Endocrinologist**
  - A pediatrician who specializes in diabetes and has the experience to care for children, adolescents, and young adults with diabetes. At Joslin, your child will usually see the endocrinologist every 6 months.
- **Nurse Educator/Nurse Practitioners**
  - A nurse that helps you and your child gain the necessary skills to manage diabetes and any related issues. At Joslin, your child will see the nurse educator every 6 months alternating with visits to your endocrinologist.
- **Dietitian**
  - A registered dietitian (RD) is an expert in food and nutrition. The RD can help you and your child select healthy food choices and develop meal plans that optimize your child's growth while maintaining blood glucose levels in your child's blood glucose target range. You and your child will see the dietitian once or twice a year.
- **Exercise Physiologist**
  - An exercise physiologist is an expert in physical activity and exercise. An exercise physiologist will help you and your child develop an age-appropriate individualized exercise plan.
- **Psychologist/Social Worker**
  - The diagnosis of diabetes in your child, as well as the continuing life needs of a person with diabetes, can be difficult for families, as the condition affects every aspect of your child's life and, thus, your own. A social worker and/or psychologist can provide support and encouragement to help families deal with the diagnosis of diabetes and how it affects the child and his or her family.
- **Child Life Specialist**
  - A child life specialist focuses on helping your child cope with the daily realities of diabetes as appropriate to your child's developmental level. Child life specialists at Joslin provide support during procedures and will work with you and your son or daughter to promote appropriate coping

strategies. During your child's clinic visits there is usually a child life specialist available to lead activities involving your child so that you can focus on learning about your child's care.

- **Ophthalmologist/Optometrist**
  - Children with diabetes should have their eyes examined by an ophthalmologist or an optometrist after 3 to 5 years of having diabetes or at puberty, whichever comes first, and yearly thereafter.
- **Pediatrician/Primary Care Provider**
  - Your child's pediatrician or other primary care provider will continue to care for your child's routine healthcare needs, including regular immunizations. Since diabetes may affect many aspects of your child's routine medical care, you, your child's primary care provider, and your diabetes team members will work closely together.
- **School Nurse and other school personnel**
  - Since your child spends much of his or her waking hours in school, members of the school staff, including school nurses, coaches, teachers, secretaries, and cafeteria staff are also important components of your child's team. The School Nurse will coordinate the school diabetes healthcare team.

Diabetes Treatment Goals

Joslin Clinic's approach to diabetes management is based upon the need to provide insulin therapy in a manner that most closely matches the way in which the body's pancreas produces and releases insulin in response to carbohydrates in the meal plan. The goals of therapy are based upon a very important study called the Diabetes Control and Complications Trial (DCCT). This critical study proved that efforts to normalize blood glucose levels using intensive insulin therapy reduces the risk for long-term complications involving the eyes, kidneys, nerves, and heart. We check for the success of therapy using a blood test obtained in the health-care professional's office, clinic, or hospital (not in the home) called a

Table 2-1. Age-Specific Blood Glucose and A1C Goals

Age (years)	Blood Glucose Goal Range (mg/dL)		A1C
	Before Meals	Bedtime/Overnight	
Toddlers and Preschoolers (0–6)	100–180 mg/dL	110–200 mg/dL	<8.5%
School age (6–12)	90–180 mg/dL	100–180 mg/dL	<8.0%
Adolescents and Young adults (13–19)	90–130 mg/dL	90–150 mg/dL	<7.5%
Adults (19+)	70–130 mg/dL	70–130 mg/dL	<7.0%

hemoglobin A1C — often referred to as just A1C. Chapter 6: Monitoring Glucose and Ketones, details the meaning of the A1C. Our team approach to care uses daily blood glucose levels along with the A1C measure as a means to determine if diabetes treatment needs to change. A1C goals are age-specific and appear in Table 2-1.

Diabetes Education

Diabetes is a long-term and complex condition which requires complicated medical management. Survival education, the basic education necessary for you and your child at diagnosis, is followed by ongoing education. To provide quality care, many members of the multidisciplinary team, and in particular the pediatric diabetes nurse educator, dietitian, and doctor, are needed as diabetes management is a continuous process that must evolve as a child grows and develops. Medical management of diabetes includes:

- Frequent blood glucose monitoring
- Timely administration of insulin
- Provision of meals and snacks
- An exercise program which is both therapeutic and recreational

The process of educating family and children about the details of management and diabetes care in general, begins at the time of diagnosis and proceeds across the life-span. At diagnosis, children and family members are often overwhelmed and are thus unable to comprehend the full spectrum of information needed to manage the child's diabetes at home. To ensure that families learn all that they need, ongoing family management training continues after diagnosis and throughout the stages of childhood and adolescence. Initially, the young child often is the bystander for diabetes education while the parents learn the approaches to diabetes management. The young child needs only to cooperate with the administration of insulin and the monitoring of blood glucose and ketone levels by caring adults. The young child will follow the behaviors and patterns of his or her parents and family members regarding healthy eating and physical activity. As the child enters school, he or she begins to take on a greater part of the diabetes management program, at times by assisting with checking blood glucose levels, although the school-age youth would not be expected to interpret the results and determine therapy. As children enter the middle and high school years, they accept greater responsibility for their diabetes self-management.

Goals of Diabetes Education

Diabetes education is key to blood glucose control. It empowers families with children with diabetes by instilling knowledge and confidence through a variety of practices that can be used at different stages of a child's life. As diabetes education involves the care of young children, school-aged children, and adolescents, parents' participation is essential; they may often be viewed as patients as well. However, as your child ages, he or she will be encouraged to share, when appropriate, responsibilities for his or her glucose control.

In spite of the tremendous advancements made in the treatment of diabetes, education is the most important tool in diabetes control. Since there are many variables that affect blood glucose levels such as food, exercise, illness, stress, and injury, education provides a crucial tool to help achieve blood glucose control. Further, education can help to promote the optimal growth and development of children and reduce the risk of complications related to diabetes. Additionally, as part of the education process, your diabetes healthcare team will assist in communicating your child's needs to schools as well as helping to keep the stress of diabetes as low as possible within the family.

Table 2-2. Pediatric & Adolescent Diabetes Education Content Areas	
Defining Diabetes	Diabetes supplies
Tools of Diabetes Management	Management of hypoglycemia
Types of insulin	Management of hyperglycemia
Insulin administration	Management of Sick Days
Oral medication administration	Physical activity and play
Blood glucose goals	Nutrition
Blood glucose monitoring	Growth and development
Ketone monitoring	Family issues

To be effective, diabetes education must be individualized based on your child's age at diagnosis and his or her current age and developmental stage. The family and the child are encouraged to ask questions during all clinical visits. The child's questions will be answered in an age-appropriate manner. The specific content areas addressed during initial and ongoing pediatric and adolescent diabetes education are shown in Table 2-2.

The objectives of diabetes education are to have families gain the ability to:

- Balance insulin/oral medication with food intake and physical activity
- Maintain normal physical growth and development
- Follow the principles of healthy nutrition as taught and individualized by a registered dietitian
- Use the results of finger stick blood glucose monitoring to:
  - safely and effectively predict needs (insulin dosage, oral medication dosage, food requirements)
  - react to changes (exercise, illness, injury)
  - provide flexibility
- Learn the methods of adjusting insulin doses

As part of your education you will be given written guidelines and suggested literature for review. As already stated, adult family members are responsible for the child's day-to-day diabetes management. These management tasks include the following:

- Keeping track of diabetes supplies
- Communicating with school personnel
- Ensuring that correct insulin doses or oral medication doses are administered at the right time
- Making certain that blood glucose levels are routinely checked and reviewed
- Communicating with your healthcare team when blood glucose readings are out of target range or during crisis situations

Visit Frequency

Your healthcare team will help you decide how often and when you and your child need to have medical and nutrition visits as well as frequency of support visits. When everything is new, these visits might occur every few weeks. As your confidence level grows (and it will!) the visits will be spaced further apart. At other times, such as during rapid growth periods, the visits may again occur at more frequent intervals. The American Diabetes Association standard of care for follow-up is for quarterly visits at a minimum. Nutrition diabetes education and update should occur 1-2 times per year as determined by your child's growth, height and weight, appetite, activity changes, and your questions. You will be able to contact your healthcare team between office visits to ask questions, review blood glucose results, support you and your child through illness and infection, and problem solve situations as they occur. Your healthcare team is only a phone call away. Remember to keep the phone numbers of your healthcare team handy and make sure to call them if your child is experiencing any of the following emergencies:

- Vomiting
- Blood glucose levels over 350
- Positive ketones
- Situations that must be managed before the next work day to ensure your child's safety

Tools of Diabetes Management: An Overview

Insulin

Your first and most immediate priority is learning how to draw up insulin into a syringe and administer it. Learning to administer insulin is not a choice but a necessity. Your child must have insulin to survive. Injected insulin replaces what the pancreas is no longer producing. You will be supported by your healthcare team who will demonstrate and practice with you until you can do it accurately. You may feel you are all thumbs when you start but with practice you will become more comfortable. Your healthcare team will decide whether you need to learn how to draw up one kind of insulin in the syringe (a single dose) or whether you need to learn how to mix 2 kinds together (a mixed dose). They will also teach you how to administer insulin and where to inject. Your nurse educator may give you an injection of saline (salt water) or ask you to give it to yourself. Parents are frequently surprised and relieved to experience what an insulin injection feels like. For many parents, their experience with injections is that of a flu or tetanus vaccination. Those injections may hurt as they are injections with larger needles into a muscle; but insulin is injected into fatty tissue with a needle so thin that there is less discomfort. To learn more about insulin, read Chapter 4: Insulin.

Blood Glucose Monitoring

You and your child are invaluable members of the diabetes management team. Part of your work will be to provide information to the healthcare team about the effectiveness of your child's insulin, meal, and exercise plans. This feedback is the result of you or your child checking blood glucose levels. Blood glucose levels provide the "roadmap" to guide safe and effective diabetes management for you and your child. To check blood glucose you'll need the following items:

- A blood glucose meter
- Blood glucose strips specific to that meter
- Lancets
- A lancing device

Your healthcare team will help you select the meter most appropriate for you and your child. Blood glucose checks help you and your healthcare team to make decisions about insulin doses, determine a need to treat blood glucose immediately if it is too low or too high, and decide whether an additional snack should be eaten before, during, or after an activity. Blood glucose checks are done before and sometimes after meals, at bedtime, and if there are symptoms of a low or high blood glucose. It is not unusual for blood glucose levels to be checked every two hours during the day. You will also be taught how and when to check for blood or urine ketones, which are by-products of your body burning fat for energy when it does not have enough insulin available. Keeping a written record or logbook of these blood glucose and ketone readings will help you and your healthcare team makes the best decisions about your child's care. Your diabetes management team cannot do it without your help! To learn more about monitoring, read Chapter 6: Monitoring Glucose and Ketones.

Meal Planning – Medical Nutrition Therapy

You will meet with a pediatric registered dietitian who will teach you how to choose healthy foods, count carbohydrates, and read and interpret food labels. You will work together to keep meals and snacks healthy, fun, and interesting. Your child's meal plan will be carefully constructed to blend in with school and home meal times, as well as family and individual food preferences. Children with diabetes do eat fast food, go to birthday parties, and participate in holiday events. Meal planning does not mean a restrictive diet, but rather a heart-healthy meal plan that meets your child's nutritional needs for growth, development, and living well. Additionally, it should lead to optimal glycemic control, lipid levels and fitness leading to overall diabetes management. To learn more about nutrition and meal planning see Chapter 7: Healthy Eating and Nutrition.

Physical Activity

Physical activity is a very important part of a healthy lifestyle and should be fun for you and your child. The child with diabetes benefits from physical activity just like his or her peers without diabetes and the rest of your family. Well-controlled or managed diabetes allows children to participate in any activity of their choosing and they are able to play just as much and as hard as they did before diabetes. Signing up for a sport or activity or getting a family membership to the local health club is a good idea for everyone in the family. Participating in physical activity through taking a dance class, gymnastics, martial arts, basketball, soccer, etc., benefits muscle strength, weight, blood glucose values, and emotional health as well. Go for it! To learn more about physical activity and its effects on diabetes read Chapter 8: Physical Activity and Diabetes Management.

Diabetes Lab Tests

With almost every medical appointment you should anticipate that there will be a trip to the phlebotomy lab for a finger stick (like a finger stick that you do when you check your blood glucose). The lab test that will be done with each visit is called an A1C (also called a glycohemoglobin or hemoglobin A1C). To learn more about the A1C test, see Chapter 6: Monitoring Glucose and Ketones.

Annually, you should anticipate a need for an arm (venous) blood draw. There are some blood tests that need more than a drop of blood. You can ask to be included in the timing of that blood draw so that you can be prepared to support your child through this procedure. Some children benefit from the use of a numbing cream or spray applied to the arm before the procedure. If you know that the visit is going to include an arm draw, ask for the numbing cream to be applied when you first come in for your visit.

Other common blood tests may be done to evaluate:

- Thyroid function
- Lipid levels
- Screening for celiac disease

Your child may be asked to give a urine sample to check for ketones and/or protein. Again, your healthcare team will explain what tests are ordered and why, as well as ensure that both you and your primary care provider will be informed of the results.

Your child is unique and wonderful and will grow and develop like any other child into a vibrant member of her or his community. Participating in any activities she or he desires, such as clubs, sports, parties, homework, and playing with friends, are all part of the world to which your child belongs. Diabetes does not restrict children from activities to which they look forward, such as class trips, vacations, and day and overnight camps.

Children with diabetes are not immune from well-child care needs such as regular check-ups, immunizations, dental work, etc., as well as childhood infections and illnesses. In fact, since illnesses and infections adversely affect diabetes, it is vitally important not to neglect general health issues due to sole concentration on diabetes. Additionally, when you are feeling alone and overwhelmed with all the tasks related to diabetes management, the behavioral and mental health specialists are important resources for you and your child.

You don't have to manage diabetes alone. It is very important that you work with a healthcare team that is knowledgeable about pediatric diabetes and can provide the support that you, your child, and the rest of your family need. It may take time, but you and your family will adjust. The more your family learns about diabetes, the more confidence you'll gain. You'll settle into a routine in which diabetes will be just one aspect of life and not the center of family interactions. Remember, your healthcare team's goal is the same as your own: for your child to be happy, healthy, successful, and maintain normal growth and development while looking toward a productive and complication-free future. Diabetes needs to fit into the family's lifestyle, not control it.

References and Resources

Butler, Deborah A., Lawlor, Margaret T., It Takes a Village: Helping Families Live With Diabetes. *Diabetes Spectr*. 2004; 17: 26-31

Silverstein J, Klingensmith G, Copeland K, Plotnick L, Kaufman F, Laffel L et al. Care of children and adolescents with type 1 diabetes: a statement of the American Diabetes Association. *Diabetes Care*. 2005; 28(1):186-212.

Lawlor M, Laffel L, Anderson B, Bertorelli A. *Caring for Young Children Living with Diabetes: Professional Manual*. Boston, MA: Joslin Diabetes Center, 1996.

Lawlor MT, Laffel L, Anderson BJ. *Blood Sugar Monitoring Owner's Manual*. Boston, MA: Joslin Diabetes Center, 1997.

Web sites:

- Joslin Diabetes Center: www.joslin.org
- American Diabetes Association: www.diabetes.org
- Children with Diabetes: www.childrenwithdiabetes.com

3

Growth and Development: The Ages and Stages

This chapter will highlight the details of the developmental stages and the expectations as children progress through normal growth and development, puberty, and traverse from childhood into adolescence and young adulthood. Just like the growing child without diabetes, the child with diabetes should enjoy normal growth and development and be faced with the usual psychosocial and behavioral trials and tribulations of each stage of development. However, the addition of diabetes to the period of pubertal growth and development may yield other challenges that we can anticipate and manage, as covered later in this book.

Child Growth and Development

You and your diabetes team share the common goal of managing diabetes in a way that promotes your child's current well-being and prevents future risk while, at the same time, allowing for the continuation of healthy growth and development. A young person with diabetes must achieve the same developmental milestones as a peer who does not have diabetes in order to become a successful adult. As a parent or other primary caretaker of a child with diabetes, you perform a daily balancing act between being present to carefully manage blood glucose levels to allow for his or her full participation in school, sports, and other activities and progressively blending into the background as he or she seeks more independent experience in the world.

Your child's response to living with diabetes will depend on many factors. Developmental stage, individual temperament, age at diagnosis, health beliefs and other attitudes of other family members and peers, and cultural expectations all contribute to how your child thinks about having diabetes.

Stages of Development

Early Childhood: (1–4 years)

Middle Childhood: (5–10 years)

Early Adolescence: (10–13 years)

Middle Adolescence: (14–17 years)

Late Adolescence (17–25+ years)

From: Hagan JF, Shaw JS, Duncan PM, Eds. *Bright Futures: Guidelines for Health Supervision of Infants, Children, and Adolescents*, 3rd ed. Elk Grove Village, IL: American Academy of Pediatrics; 2008.

A child's accommodation to the ever-present diabetes management tasks will change over time as he or she views his or her world from shifting developmental perspectives. One child may adjust relatively easily to life with diabetes when first diagnosed, then be subject to angry outbursts a year or two later. Another child initially resists every insulin injection and blood glucose check, but, given time, develops into the diabetes-camp counselor who is viewed as a role model by campers and staff alike. Your school-age child may wear an insulin pump as a badge of honor, only to reject that pump as a visible sign of having diabetes when entering adolescence.

It is important to realize that no matter how your child thinks about having diabetes it will be different from the way you think about it. Young children see the world in a concrete, literal way. One poignant story told by a parent of a 6 year-old child with diabetes recounts the day when the whole family participated enthusiastically in a local "walk for a cure." At the end of the walk, the child tearfully expressed disappointment that his diabetes had not gone away.

Adolescents show increasing ability to think abstractly but remain rooted in day-to-day experience. Our expectation that an adolescent will be able to look ahead 20 years and seek to protect himself now from risk of complications in the future does not match what we have come to know about adolescent development.

Your child is unique and will develop at his or her own pace. The following are some very general guidelines as to how children and adolescents make meaning of having a special healthcare need, such as diabetes, according to developmental stage. These stages are broad and overlapping.

The American Academy of Pediatrics and Bright Futures provides these "Domains of Development" to guide you as a parent and us, your diabetes healthcare team, in understanding your child at various points along the continuum of development. Your child may show behaviors typical of more than a single age or stage or may exhibit few, if any, of the described characteristics.

Early Childhood (1–4 years): "After tomorrow I won't need to check my blood glucose again."

Very young children live in a world of magic and fantasy. In this world simply having or expressing a thought can make it happen. A young child may believe that the new onset of a condition such as diabetes is punishment for a misbehavior or negative thought. No matter what factual explanations you have shared, your young child with diabetes is likely to harbor the magical belief that he will wake up without diabetes some day in the near future.

Your young child learns words and routines through play. Children in early childhood lack the capacity to understand why the tasks of diabetes management have become a necessary part of their lives, but they can be very creative at making meaning of diabetes as they mimic their adult caretakers' words and behaviors. Those of us who have the good fortune of being able to observe and listen to children with diabetes as they participate in child life activities during clinic visits gain great respect for the little ones' abilities to let others know what diabetes means to them.

There is a broad range of normal behavior in these early years. Temperament may play a strong role in a child's response to the experiences of blood glucose checks and injections. One child may accept routines and limits readily while another resists with all of her or his might. As young children acquire socialization skills and learn to interact with other children and adults, they begin to internalize positive or negative attitudes towards themselves and others. Towards the end of this developmental period, your child may be beginning to discern differences in individuals and may question why he or she is the only one in his peer group who needs shots or finger sticks.

Intensive diabetes management, with frequent blood glucose monitoring and multiple injections or insulin pump boluses, is more common in this age group than it was just a few years ago. Your child may be more anxious about starting school than his or her peers because you may have been close by to manage his or her diabetes. At the same time, he or she may be increasingly bothered by being interrupted for diabetes management tasks because he or she is more intensely involved with activities and interactive play.

Middle Childhood (5–10 years): "I can do it myself!"

Children in middle childhood experience rapid development in the areas of general knowledge, physical abilities, and social skills. As she or he rapidly gains competence in many areas, your child will increasingly compare her or his own abilities, appearance, and daily routine to those of other children, using this information to develop a unique sense of self. Children in this age group may begin to single out or avoid peers whom they define as different. Children enter middle childhood as magical thinkers and progress to more logical approaches to understanding. Concrete, literal thinking becomes more abstract. The older school-age child acquires concepts of illness and disability that are more realistic and factually based.

It is in the later years of this developmental stage that your child may begin to take some responsibility in checking her or his own blood glucose and maybe even injecting insulin. Children can learn to perform these tasks very capably, and gaining new skills usually results in positive feedback from the important adults in a child's life. We must remember, however, that diabetes management tasks are endlessly repetitive and the result of all this work can be unpredictable and frustrating. Children in this age range and older quickly tire of being responsible for the daily tasks of diabetes management. An easy solution from the child's perspective may be to skip a blood glucose check, but report a blood glucose that is in target range. This can reflect several different reasons including, being too busy, not wanting to bring diabetes into social experiences, not wanting to do it due to diabetes fatigue, or saving face. If a child gives most of his or her own injections, he or she may forget or elect to omit an injection. He or she may put all the injections he or she does give in exactly the same site. If your child chooses to participate in diabetes care tasks such as monitoring blood glucose or injecting insulin, it is important that you directly supervise these tasks and explain that you will still be giving many of the injections and performing some of the blood glucose checks. Make sure that your child sees this as support rather than punishment. This helps your child understand that managing diabetes is an adult responsibility, freeing her or him to attend to all the other demands of normal development.

Early adolescence (10–13 years): "Everybody is looking at me. I hate my diabetes."

A child in early adolescence is inclined to magnify his or her personal situation, believing that his or her problems are unique. This may lead to loneliness and isolation. Physical appearance and blending into a social group become important driving forces of early adolescent behavior. Your young adolescent may suddenly refuse to cope with a diabetes management task such as blood glucose checking that he or she had previously been involved with. Young people who were comfortable with everyone knowing about their diabetes in elementary school may wish for far more privacy in middle or junior high school. As a young adolescent meets new friends and joins new groups, he or she may no longer share that they have diabetes. Children in this age range are developmentally unable to recognize that they are personally vulnerable to long-term complications of chronic illness. In middle childhood, a young adolescent may decide it is easier to invent a blood glucose result. This is easier than explaining that the result was high because they had an extra snack and did not want an extra injection or that they simply forgot to check. The explanation that insulin is no longer working or the dose needs to be adjusted may be that some of the injections or pump boluses were actually never given. Young adolescents who omit insulin out of forgetfulness, because they are in a hurry, or because they are embarrassed to share the fact of their diabetes with peers, can be very responsible and honest in other areas of their lives. They are signaling to us that they are not developmentally ready to be fully responsible for the complexities of diabetes management.

Middle adolescence (14–17 years): "Ask me about my day, not my diabetes."

A young person with diabetes in middle adolescence may continue to feel different and inadequate in comparison to his or her peers and may remain reluctant to perform diabetes management tasks in front of them. The amount of time an adolescent in this age range spends away from home increases. A long school day may be immediately followed by an activity requiring the adolescent to be away from home from early morning until dinnertime. Young people in this age range may continue to neglect care needed to manage diabetes but may view asking for adult help as a sign of personal failure. Adolescents live in the present and share an inability to clearly picture themselves in the future. Frustrated (and frightened) parents may resort to repeating the numerous complications of diabetes to a child who may not be listening.

Many adolescents with diabetes complain that during the few daily opportunities to talk with a parent, they are peppered with questions about their diabetes while, at the same time, a sibling without diabetes is asked about school and extracurricular activities. You may find that it works better to schedule a regular time to sit down with your teenager to review diabetes management, including a review of the glucose meter memory or pump history, so that when they first walk through the door, or during dinner, you can discuss other topics.

Late adolescence and Emerging Adulthood (17–25+ years): "I am starting to realize that I need to take care of my diabetes, but I am so busy with other things."

The older adolescent approaching adulthood should be experiencing increasing stability of self-esteem and comfort with a sense of self that includes diabetes. The older adolescent, in theory, begins to make more independent decisions about healthcare and starts to recognize the importance of his behavior to prevent future health risks. Therefore, the older adolescent may be more successful with diabetes management as they start to take on other responsibilities.

In reality, not all adolescents, including those with diabetes, make this transition at the same rate. Parents of older adolescents and young adults may find themselves struggling to support their child's aspirations and dreams even as they realize that diabetes management has not yet become an important priority. There may be additional problems such as depression or an eating disorder that prevent the older adolescent from assuming independence within this time frame (see Chapter 14: Behavioral Pitfalls — Prevention and Early Intervention for more information).

If your child attends college, the first year may be particularly challenging. If diabetes management tasks are not a very routine part of daily life, new social routines and academic pressures may distract your child from managing diabetes. For example, if your adolescent has been offered a sports scholarship or if they are considering a school far from home, they will have several transition issues to deal with. That is why it is so important to plan ahead with your child and see how you can support your child during this transitional period (see Chapter 17: Transitions: The Challenges of Life After High School for more information).

Even when an older adolescent appears to be making a very successful transition to adulthood, many parents find that they are able to continue to provide support without being overly intrusive. Keeping track of prescriptions, scheduling appointments, and accompanying your older adolescent to clinic visits, at least as far as the waiting room, may be appreciated. As your older adolescent becomes more independent, ask how you may be helpful and continue to express your interest in her or his diabetes along with all the other important aspects of her or his life.

Summary

Many things go into the successful management of diabetes. Having a team that incorporates both family and healthcare professionals creates an environment in which individualized care can be provided. Attention must be paid to the age, stage, and temperament of the child with diabetes as well as a variety of family characteristics.

References and Resources

Brazelton TB, Greenspan SI. *The Irreducible Needs of Children: What Every Child Must Have to Grow, Learn, and Flourish*. New York, NY: Perseus Publishing; 2000.

Dixon SD, Stein MT. *Encounters with Children: Pediatric Behavior and Development*, 3rd ed. St. Louis, MO: Mosby; 2000.

Hagan JF, Shaw JS, Duncan PM, Eds. *Bright Futures: Guidelines for Health Supervision of Infants, Children, and Adolescents*, 3rd ed. Elk Grove Village, IL: American Academy of Pediatrics; 2008.

Web sites:

- Joslin Diabetes Center: www.joslin.org
- American Diabetes Association: www.diabetes.org
- Juvenile Diabetes Research Foundation: www.jdrf.org
- American Association of Diabetes Educators: www.diabeteseducator.org
- American Academy of Pediatrics Parenting Corner: www.aap.org
- Children With Diabetes: www.childrenwithdiabetes.com
- Child Development Information on Center for Disease Control and Prevention: www.cdc.gov/ncbddd/child
- Child Development Information on Public Broadcasting System (PBS): www.pbs.org/parents

4

Insulin

Insulin is a natural hormone that plays an important role in the body's metabolism of food. When food is digested, glucose enters the blood stream. Insulin is then required to transport glucose from the blood stream into cells where it can be used for energy. Without insulin, your body is unable to utilize glucose and will create a state of malnutrition. You can think of insulin as a key that unlocks a cell to let glucose enter.

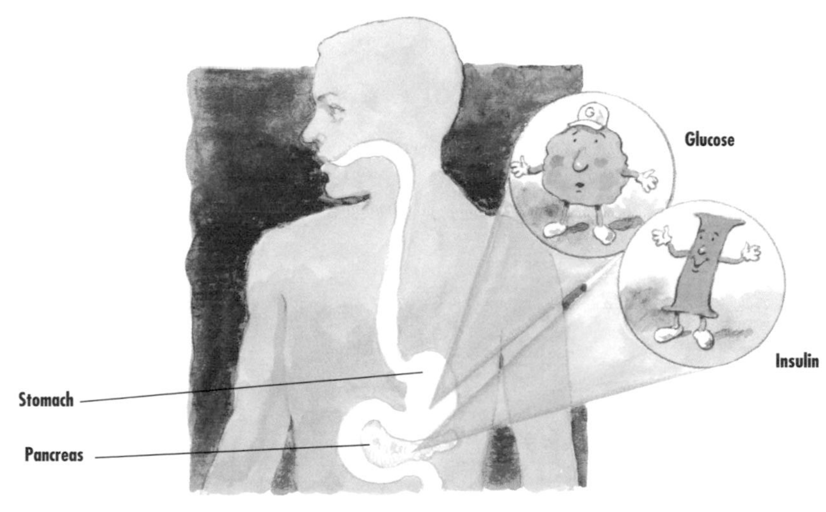

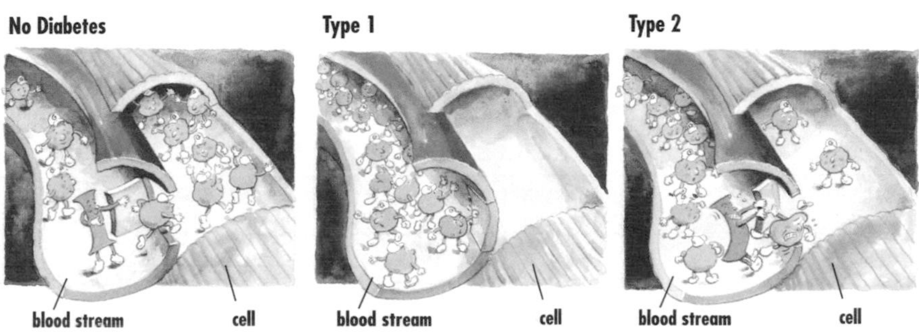

Too much glucose can be harmful. It can build up in different parts of the body like the eyes, kidneys, nerves, and heart. This can cause problems over time.

Insulin Types

Insulin is divided by the following types:

- Rapid-acting insulin (lispro, aspart, or glulisine)
- Short-acting insulin (Regular)
- Intermediate-acting insulin (NPH)
- Basal or long-acting insulin (glargine and detemir)

In addition there are a number of premixed insulins. Each of these combines 2 types of insulin.

- **Humulin / Novolin 70/30** is 70% NPH and 30% Regular, a combination of intermediate and fast acting insulin
- **Humalog Mix 50/50** is 50% insulin lispro protamine and 50% insulin lispro
- **Humalog 75/25** is 75% insulin lispro protamine and 25% insulin lispro,
- **NovoLog Mix 70/30** 70% insulin aspart protamine and 30% insulin aspart injection

Insulin Strength

The strength of insulin used in the United States is called U-100. If you are traveling internationally and need to get your insulin replaced due to lost vials or its having spoiled due to heat, extreme cold, or being beyond the expiration date, it could be possible that you are prescribed an insulin of a different strength. REMEMBER – if you are using U-100 insulin, it must be drawn up into a syringe with an ORANGE cap. If you have another strength of insulin, ask the healthcare provider to provide you with an appropriate syringe or to show you how to convert the strength to its U-100 equivalent strength.

Also available is the short-acting U-500 regular insulin with U-500 lispro soon to be available. U-500 insulin is five times stronger than U-100 insulin. Its use is very rare.

Insulin Action

Insulin is categorized based on the timing of its action, including when it starts to work (onset), when it works hardest (peak), and when it has finished working (duration). Your diabetes team will work with you to find an insulin plan that works best for your child and your family lifestyle. It is important to familiarize yourself with the timing of insulin action in order to plan meals and snacks accordingly, track blood glucose trends, and consider insulin dose adjustments. **Table 4-1** and **Figure 4-1** describe the various types of insulin in terms of their action.

It is important to note that insulin action may differ from person to person. The onset, peak, and duration of insulin may also be affected by

Table 4-1. Insulin Action

	Product	When To Take	Onset	Peak	Duration
Rapid-Acting	lispro (Humalog) aspart (Novolog) glulisine (Apidra)	0–15 min before meal	10–30 min	30 min– 3 hours	3–5 hours
Short-Acting	Regular (R) Human	30 min before meal	30–60 min	2–5 hours	Up to 12 hours
Intermediate-Acting	NPH (N) Human	Does not need to be given with meal	90 min– 4 hours	4–12 hours	Up to 24 hours
Long Acting	glargine (Lantus) detemir (Levemir)	Does not need to be given with meal	45 min– 4 hours	Minimal	Up to 24 hours

Figure 4-1. Common Insulin Regimens and their Action Curves. These graphs depict examples of common insulin regimens with the action curve for different types of insulin.

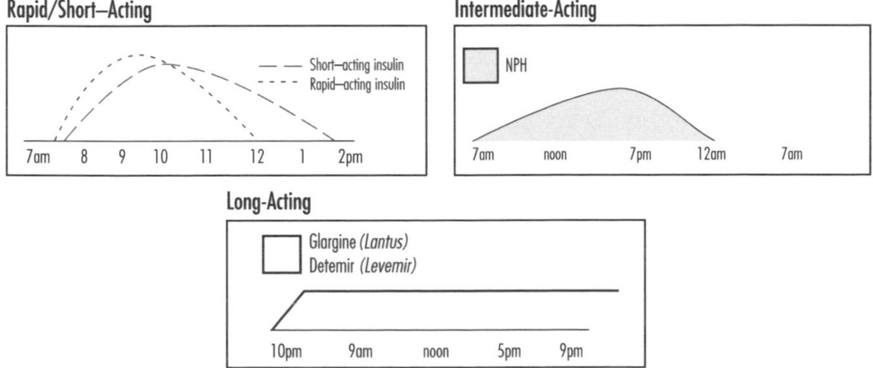

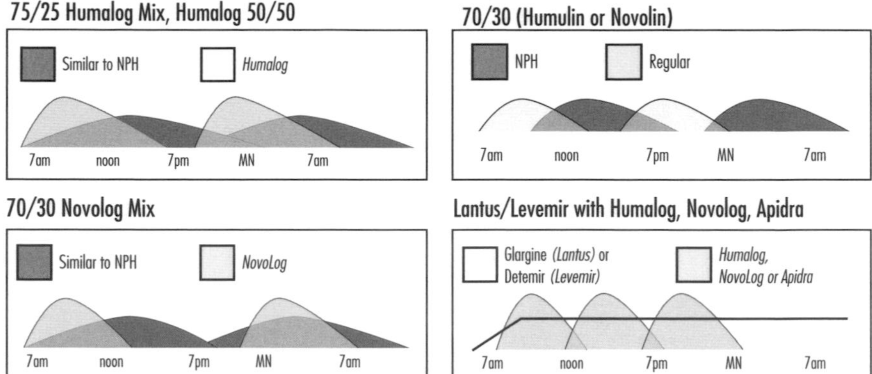

the injection site chosen, the time that the injection is given (night versus daytime), and physical activity level before or after the injection is given.

Insulin Dosing

Many factors determine the amount of insulin your child will need to keep his or her blood glucose within target range. A few of these many factors are length of time since diagnosis, age, rate of growth, and amount of regular exercise. Some parents worry that their child's need for more insulin means that the diabetes has gotten worse, but this is not the case. Among many causes for increased insulin is a drop-off in your child's ability to produce his or her own insulin if newly diagnosed, normal growth, puberty, or a decrease in accustomed activity. Like most medication, the amount of insulin your child is receiving is evaluated in terms of the total amount of insulin your child receives in a day and your child's weight in kilograms (1 kilogram = 2.2 pounds). For example, a child who weighs 66 pounds weighs 30 kilograms. If the same child is getting a total of 21 units of all types of insulin on average every day, he is receiving 0.7 units of insulin per kilogram per day. Usually when children are first diagnosed with diabetes, they require between 0.5 and 1.0 unit per kilogram per day. Often the child has an increase in his own insulin production after several weeks of receiving injected insulin (called the honeymoon phase) and in some cases may require smaller doses of long-acting insulin to maintain near normal blood glucose levels for an indefinite period of time. However, during the honeymoon period the child will always continue to receive insulin therapy. Eventually this insulin production slows, and the child's need for injected insulin increases again. As your child approaches puberty, however, it is common for insulin requirements to increase under the influence of the hormones that are associated with pubertal development. Adolescents who are experiencing rapid growth and development may require 1.5 or more units of insulin per kilogram per day to maintain blood glucose in target range.

Insulin dosing should be given before eating. There are a few situations when it may be advantageous to administer rapid-acting insulin during or immediately after eating. Busy toddlers or children who are recovering from illness may have very unpredictable appetites. In these unusual situations, it may be better to wait until your child has eaten most of the meal before calculating the insulin dose even though the peak of the rapid-acting insulin may not be as good a match for the peak in your child's blood glucose. However, after-meal insulin dosing is not appropriate for the vast number of children; insulin should be given before meals in the vast majority of circumstances.

Insulin Plans

A successful insulin plan replaces the insulin no longer produced by the beta cells of the pancreas in a way that most closely copies the body's insulin production while providing the best fit for your family's needs and capabilities. A plan that works for a child who attends a school with a full-time nurse may not be the best plan for a child who does not have access

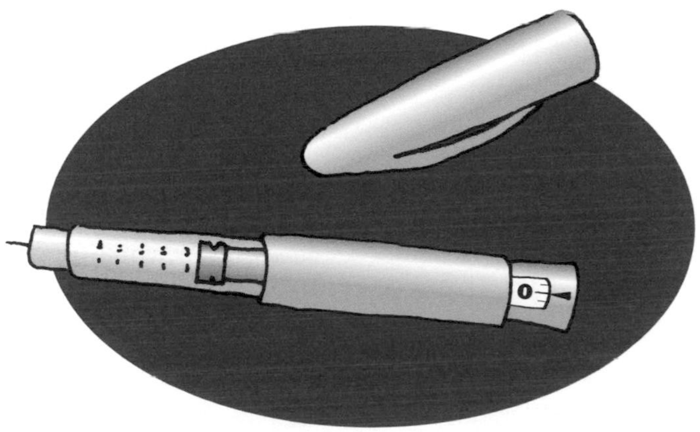

to an adult trained to manage diabetes during the school day. Injecting insulin at all meal and snack times may work beautifully when a child is closely supervised by parents and school personnel, but the same plan may be overwhelming for a child without adequate adult support.

You and your diabetes team will have many opportunities to discuss and evaluate various approaches to meeting your child's insulin needs and design the best management plan for your child's and family's needs. The plan will likely change over time with your child's growth and the impact of new schedules. Any of the following plans may be the best for your child at a particular time.

Basal/Bolus Insulin Plan

The current gold standard approach to diabetes management, called intensive management, uses a *basal/bolus* insulin plan. Insulin given in this way can be delivered either through multiple daily injections (MDI) or by means of continuous subcutaneous insulin infusion (CSII) using an insulin pump. One advantage of basal/bolus plans is the ability to be more flexible with the timing of meals and snacks and with the amount of carbohydrate eaten. This plan does not require set meal and snack times to accommodate an insulin peak. A disadvantage of basal/bolus insulin plans is the need to give an injection of insulin every time carbohydrate is eaten. The particular advantages and disadvantages of CSII are discussed in Chapter 5: Insulin Pumps.

A basal/bolus plan uses long-acting insulin, insulin detemir (Levemir) or insulin glargine (Lantus) in 1-2 daily injections to meet your child's background or *basal* insulin need. Additional injections of rapid-acting insulin, *bolus* insulin, are given before meals and snacks in amounts calculated to cover the amount of carbohydrate being eaten and to correct elevated blood glucose as needed. You will be taught how to calculate these bolus injections using an *insulin-to-carbohydrate ratio* which is the number of grams of carbohydrate a single unit of insulin covers. You will also be taught to use a *correction* or *sensitivity factor* which is the number of points (mg/dL) of blood glucose a single unit of insulin will decrease the blood glucose. Finally, you and your diabetes team will select a *target blood glucose* goal. These calculations may seem difficult at first, but once you get used to them, they are easy to use. We recommend that you be

Table 4-2. Basal/Bolus — Common Terms

Basal insulin — The insulin that controls blood glucose levels between meals and overnight. It controls glucose in the fasting state. The basal insulin is provided as the basal rate by a pump or as the long-acting insulin injected by syringe or pen. Basal insulin is generally half of the total daily insulin dose.

Basal/bolus therapy — Refers to a specific kind of physiologic insulin replacement in which basal insulin is provided with a long-acting insulin analog and bolus insulin is provided with a rapid-acting insulin analog aimed at covering elevated blood glucoses and the carbohydrates contained in meals and snacks. Treatment via an insulin pump may also be referred to in this way.

Bolus — A dose of insulin given in addition to the basal insulin to either correct a high blood glucose and/or cover carbs at a meal or snack.

Bolus insulin — The insulin that is released when food is eaten. A **bolus** is a burst of insulin that is delivered by injection or by the insulin pump to cover a meal or snack or to correct for a high blood glucose level.

Carbohydrate counting — A meal planning method commonly used by people with diabetes to plan their food and meal choices. Carbohydrate counting helps one achieve a balance between the amount of carbohydrate foods eaten and the available insulin.

CSII — Continuous subcutaneous insulin infusion, otherwise known as pump therapy.

Correction factor (CF) — A term used for the insulin dosage required to lower blood glucose to a specified target level. Correction levels are often used for patients receiving insulin pump therapy or basal/bolus multiple injection therapy. A correction factor of 1 to 50 means 1 unit of insulin will drop a blood glucose 50 points. The correction factor is also called the sensitivity index (SI). Correction factors usually vary person-to-person and even throughout the day.

Insulin pump — A small battery-powered insulin delivery system; a mechanical device, typically the size of a beeper or small cell phone that releases insulin into the tissues of the body by way of tubing and a needle.

Insulin sensitivity factor (also called the correction factor or supplemental factor) — The amount of blood glucose measured in mg/dL that is lowered by 1 unit of rapid-acting or regular insulin. The insulin sensitivity factor is used to calculate the amount of insulin needed to return blood glucose to within your target blood glucose range.

Insulin-to-Carbohydrate Ratio (I:Carb) — A method of determining how much rapid-acting insulin is needed to cover the carbohydrate eaten at a meal or snack. This is used as part of a more advanced level of carbohydrate counting.

Sensitivity Factor (also called the correction factor) — The number of points (mg/dL) the blood glucose will drop after 1 unit of insulin is given.

proficient in carbohydrate counting and meet with a diabetes educator for instruction and practice before you start this type of insulin plan.

An insulin pump uses the same approach as a basal/bolus plan with multiple injections, but the insulin is pumped through a tiny tube or catheter, *infusion set*, placed just under the skin. An insulin pump uses only rapid- or short-acting insulin. A tiny amount of this insulin, the *basal* insulin, flows through the infusion set around the clock. When it is time for a meal or snack or if blood glucose is elevated above the target level, you direct the pump to give a *bolus* using ratios that have been programmed into the pump. The pump does not do it alone!

Modified Basal/Bolus Insulin Plan

If there is no safe or practical way for your child to receive insulin at school to cover a morning snack and lunch, adding peaking intermediate-acting insulin, NPH (Humulin N or Novolin N), to the rapid-acting insulin at breakfast may allow for reasonable coverage of morning snack and lunch. The amount of long-acting insulin is reduced to account for the additional units of intermediate-acting insulin. When using this modified basal/bolus plan, you may find that the mid-afternoon snack is not sufficiently covered. An injection of rapid-acting insulin at snack time may be needed to keep your child's blood glucose in target range during the late afternoon hours.

Sliding Scale Insulin Plan

If you are using a meal plan that specifies a fixed amount of grams of carbohydrate to eat at each meal, a sliding scale can be a relatively simple way for you to figure out how much insulin to give according to your child's blood glucose and which meal is being eaten. The scale takes into account how much insulin is needed to cover the grams of carbohydrate allowed for the meal and how much it will take to bring elevated blood glucose down to target level. The set scale increases the amount of insulin for each meal as the blood glucose goes up, allowing you to correct for higher blood glucose.

For instance, if your child's meal plan allows 60 grams of carbohydrate for breakfast and your diabetes team has estimated that a unit of insulin covers 30 grams of carbohydrate, your child will need 2 units to cover breakfast as long as the blood glucose is in target range. If the blood glucose level is elevated, however, additional insulin will be required to

Table 4-3. Example of Sample Sliding Scale Insulin Plan

Breakfast: 60 grams carbohydrate	
Blood glucose level	**Units of insulin (insulin type specified)**
0–70 mg/dL	2.0 after treating for low blood glucose
71–150	2.0
151–200	2.5
201–250	3.0
251–300	3.5
301–350	4.0
351–400	4.5
over 400	5.0
(This is not to be used for dosing your child as this may either be too little or too much insulin for your child. Your healthcare team will design a sliding scale specific to your child's needs.)	

bring the level down. Supposing that the diabetes team estimates that a unit of insulin brings your child's blood glucose down about 100 points (or a ½ unit reduces the blood glucose by about 50 points), the breakfast sliding scale might look like Table 4-3.

Since a sliding scale does not meet your child's background or *basal* insulin needs, long-acting insulin, intermediate-acting insulin or both must be given as well. Insulin detemir (Levemir) or insulin glargine (Lantus) cannot be mixed with other types of insulin. They are given in separate injections due to the changes in their insulin action profile when mixed. Studies are underway to evaluate the impact of mixed dosing. However, when mixed, the immediate effect with rapid analogs is to lower the glucose level. It is possible to mix intermediate-acting insulin with rapid- or short-acting insulin to reduce the number of injections. We recommend mixing insulins produced by the same manufacturer in this case. We will discuss how to mix insulins in a later section.

If long-acting insulin such as detemir or glargine is used with a sliding scale, there will be a scale for breakfast, lunch, dinner, and snacks larger than 10-15 grams of carbohydrate. This plan is similar to the basal/bolus plan already discussed except that the meal plan is fixed. A minimum of 4 insulin injections are required with additional injections as needed for snacks.

Intensive insulin plans with multiple daily injections may be overwhelming for you and your child. Often when a child is newly diagnosed with type 1 diabetes and has some beta cells which are continuing to produce insulin, multiple injections are not yet necessary to maintain blood glucose levels in target range. Rarely, your diabetes team may recommend a plan for your child that consists of only 2-3 injections on a temporary basis. Extremely rarely, there may be a strong honeymoon phase with very young diagnosis when a child may only need a single injection of long-acting insulin, because there are enough working beta cells to meet the mealtime demands.

During the honeymoon phase, many children continue to use an insulin plan requiring three injections daily. Rapid-acting and intermediate-acting insulin are combined in a single injection before breakfast. Rapid-acting insulin is given before dinner, and a smaller dose of intermediate or long-acting insulin is given at about 9 PM to provide for the child's overnight insulin needs. There is concern with the use of intermediate-acting insulin at bedtime since there is a greater chance of overnight hypoglycemia (low blood glucose) than there is with long-acting insulin.

Pre-mixed Insulin

Some insulin comes in a pre-mixed form in which intermediate-acting insulin is already combined with a predetermined percentage of short- or rapid-acting insulin. Pre-mixed insulin is usually given 2-3 times daily, prior to meals. Pre-mixed insulin may be an option for a family that has to cope with additional stress or an adolescent who is suffering from diabetes burnout and struggling to keep up with all the tasks necessary to manage diabetes. Using pre-mixed insulin does not allow for "fine-tuning" either the rapid, short, or intermediate acting insulin as the ratio is "fixed" with the vial or cartridge.

Dilute Insulin

Some very small children and some children who have continuing beta cell function during the honeymoon phase require amounts of insulin that are

Table 4-4. Dilution Ratios to Create U-10, U-25 and U-50 Insulin			
Dilution	Parts U-100 Insulin	Parts Diluent	Units insulin per line a 30 U insulin syringe (100 u/ml)
U-10	1	9	0.1
U-25	1	3	0.25
U-50	1	1	0.5

too small to be drawn up reliably even in a syringe marked for half units. A diluting liquid, *diluent,* is available for Humulin N, Humulin R, Humalog and Novolog insulins. Generally it is the rapid-acting insulin that requires dilution. The most common dilutions are U-10, U-25 and U-50.

If your child will benefit from diluted insulin, your diabetes team will give you clear instructions, verbally and printed, and demonstrate the procedure to you. Some pharmacies will dilute insulin preparations for you.

Drawing Up Insulin

In order to deliver the correct dose of insulin it is important to know how to draw up insulin into a syringe. Table 4-5 provides steps to follow to successfully accomplish drawing up one type of insulin into a syringe.

Table 4-5. Procedure for Drawing Up a Single Insulin Dose

To draw up:

1. Wipe off the top of the bottle with an alcohol swab.
2. If the insulin is cloudy turn the bottle on its side and roll between your hands.
3. Pull plunger back to fill syringe with________ units of air.
4. With bottle flat on table, put needle through the top of the bottle and push plunger down.
5. Leave needle in the bottle and turn the bottle upside down.
6. Pull plunger halfway down to fill the syringe with insulin. Check for air bubbles. If there are no air bubbles push plunger to _____ units. If there are bubbles, push all the insulin back into the bottle. Pull plunger down again to ______ units. When there are no bubbles take needle out.

Procedure for Drawing Up a Mixed Insulin Dose

If your child is on a mixed dose of NPH and lispro, aspart or glulisine, the 2 types of insulin may be mixed in a syringe. **REMEMBER – neither detemir (Levimir) nor glargine (Lantus) can be mixed with another type of insulin. If using a syringe to draw up detemir (Levimir) or glargine (Lantus) you will always use the above instructions for drawing up a single dose.** When drawing up a mixed insulin dose in the same syringe, it is possible that very tiny amounts of the first insulin drawn up may cling to the needle and when the needle is inserted into the second vial it allows for some of that insulin to be introduced into the second vial. If this is repeated a number of times, the action pattern of the insulin in the second bottle may be altered. The principle that underlies drawing up a mixed insulin dose is that the first insulin to be drawn up into the syringe is the most rapid-acting insulin. For example, if you are mixing insulin aspart (Novolog) with NPH (Novolin N) or insulin lispro (Humalog) with NPH (Humulin N), you would draw the aspart or lispro into the syringe first and then the NPH. If you were mixing Regular

Table 4-6. Procedure for Drawing Up a Mixed Insulin Dose

To draw up:

1. Wipe off the top of the bottle with an alcohol swab and turn the **cloudy** bottle on its side to roll between your hands, for 20 seconds.
2. Pull plunger back to fill the syringe with ________ units of air. Put needle through the top of the **cloudy** bottle, keeping bottle upright on table and push plunger down putting air into bottle. Take needle out empty.
3. Pull plunger back to fill with ________ units of air. Put needle through the top of the **clear** bottle. Keeping bottle upright on table, push plunger down.
4. Leave needle in **clear** bottle and turn bottle upside down.
5. Pull plunger halfway down to fill syringe with insulin. Check for air bubbles. If there are no air bubbles push plunger to ______ units. If there are bubbles, push all the insulin back into the bottle. Pull plunger down again to _______ units. When there are no bubbles take needle out.
6. Put needle through the top of cloudy bottle and turn it upside down.
7. Pull plunger slowly to _________units. (_________+_________). Take out needle.
8. Check that you have the right number of units. If you pull up too much insulin, or if you see air bubbles, discard the insulin into the sink and go back to step 2.

insulin into the syringe in addition to the above, it would be drawn up after the aspart or lispro, but before the NPH. Table 4-6 provides steps to follow to successfully accomplish drawing up one type of insulin into a syringe.

Injection Site Selection and Rotation

The next step is selecting a site to inject the insulin. Insulin is injected into the fatty tissue just below the skin, or *subcutaneously*. There are five approved areas of insulin injection: abdomen, back of arms, front of thighs, hips, buttocks area (see Figure 4-2). You should not inject insulin into muscular areas or areas naturally prone to pressure such as the backs of thighs or lower portions of the buttocks.

Many small children do not have much fat in these areas, so your child may rotate among 2-3 of these sites instead of all 5. If injections are not carefully rotated and insulin is always given in the same locations, a condition called *lipohypertrophy* may result. Lipo refers to fat, and hypertrophy signifies exaggerated growth. Repeated injections of insulin into the same

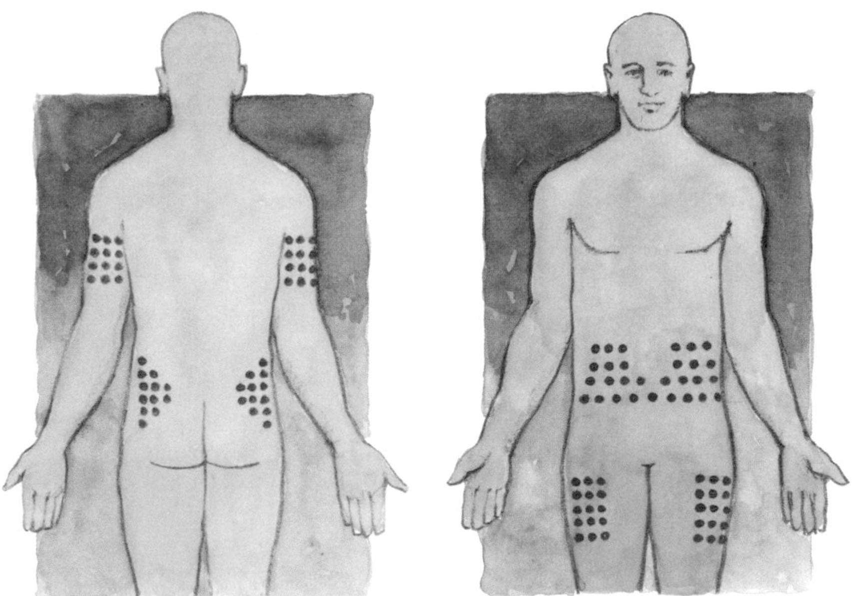

Figure 4-2. Insulin Injection Sites

Table 4-7. Procedure for Injecting Insulin

1. Chose an injection site that does not show signs of overuse such as fullness, firmness, or bruising.
2. Clean the skin with an alcohol wipe.
3. Pull up a gentle pinch of skin.
4. Holding the pinch, pick up the syringe or insulin pen like a pencil and hold it at right angles to the pinched skin.
5. Push the needle straight into the skin unless you have been instructed differently by your diabetes team.
6. Push down steadily on the syringe or insulin pen plunger until all the insulin is delivered.
7. Release the pinched skin and wait for five to ten seconds (counting helps).
8. Withdraw the needle. Observe for any leak back of insulin.
9. If the site is bleeding, apply gentle pressure with a clean tissue or piece of gauze until bleeding has stopped.

site cause an exaggerated growth of fat under the skin. These areas can be felt or even seen as lumpy, full, or thickened areas just under the skin. Insulin injected into a site that has hypertrophy is absorbed into the body less consistently than when it is injected into a healthy area. This makes the insulin action more difficult to predict. It can take several months of not using the injection site with hypertrophy to return to a more normal state, but it will.

A more unusual response to insulin injections is *lipoatrophy*. Atrophy refers to a wasting away of tissue. In this case, repeated insulin injection cause a wasting away of fat under the skin. These areas are visible as large dimples or hollows at the injection site and occasionally even at sites distant from injections. Lipoatrophy is less common since the development of the more purified human insulin and insulin analogs, but it still occurs in some individuals. Lipoatrophy does not usually go away with lack of use, but a specific type of skin cream (a prescription is required by your doctor or nurse practitioner) has shown promise in causing these areas to fill in. Consult with your diabetes care team if you notice these areas.

After you have drawn up the insulin – either the single or mixed dose – and chosen your injection site it is time to inject the insulin. Table 4-7 outlines the steps to giving the injection.

Insulin Storage

When you receive insulin from the pharmacy or through your mail order prescription service, it should be kept cool and placed in the refrigerator as soon as possible. If the insulin has been shipped to you, it should be specially packaged to keep it cool. If the insulin does not feel cool to the touch, you should notify your mail order pharmacy and consider discarding it.

A few more cautions:

- Insulin in an insulin pen form or Novolin InnoLet device should be discarded after 14 days.
- Pre-mixed insulin pens should be discarded after 10 days.
- Diluted aspart (Novolog) or lispro (Humalog), the mixed diluted insulin can be kept in the refrigerator for 28 days.
- Open insulin vials and pens should be kept between the temperatures of 59°F – 86°F.
- Whenever you begin a new type of insulin, it is important to ask your diabetes team or check the package for storage instructions so that you are not administering insulin that has lost its effectiveness.

How is Insulin Stored?

- Unopened bottles of insulin should be stored in the refrigerator and are good until the expiration date on the box and/or the bottle.
- Insulin can be stored at room temperature (59°F–86°F) for about 1 month (28–30 days or 42 days for detemir). The strength of the insulin may be altered after that.
- Date your vials or cartridges.
- Insulin should never be frozen.
- Keep insulin bottle(s) away from direct sunlight or heat and in a cool, dry place.
- Avoid exposing the bottles to temperature extremes (less than 36° or more than 86°).

References and Resources

Lopez, X, Castells, M, Ricker, A, Velazquez, EF, Mun, E, Goldfine, AB. Human insulin analog-induced lipoatrophy. *Diabetes Care*. 2008; 31:442-444.

Insulin administration. *Diabetes* Care. 2004; 27 Suppl 1:S106-S109.

Web sites:

- Eli Lilly: www.lillydiabetes.com
- Novo Nordisk: http://www.novonordisk-us.com
- Sanofi Aventis: http://www.apidra.com
- Lantus: http://www.lantus.com
- American Diabetes Association 2009 Resources Guide: http://forecast.diabetes.org
- FDA: www.fda.gov
- Guidelines for Insulin Management of Diabetes in School: ndep.nih.gov/resources

5

Insulin Pumps

Pumps, pods, basal rates, boluses, infusion sets, sensitivity factors, combination wave boluses . . . the list goes on and on; and if you are among the families considering pump therapy, it may be enough to make your head spin. Whether you and your family are new to diabetes, or well seasoned, chances are you have at least heard these terms used. Insulin pump technology has evolved tremendously in recent years, and continues to do so at a rapid pace. Injection therapy, even basal/bolus programs, requires a more structured schedule than pump therapy (also called CSII – continuous subcutaneous insulin infusion). Pump therapy offers flexibility and precision, attracting many children and teens living with diabetes to choose pump therapy as a way to manage their diabetes. Keep in mind, though, that insulin pump therapy is not for everyone; it is a great tool for many, but not all.

Although this chapter provides basic information about pump therapy, it is by no means an all-inclusive guide. There are some basics you need to

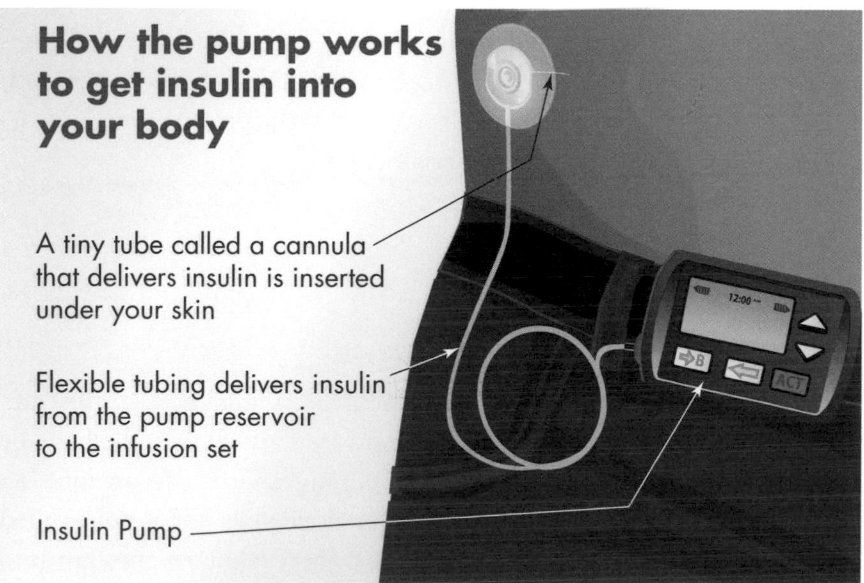

cover when beginning to consider pump therapy, and even more basics to learn when starting on an insulin pump. Much of the learning, however, is a gradual process that occurs over time. This chapter will address a basic overview of pump therapy:

- What is an insulin pump?
- How does it work?
- What is involved in starting and managing therapy?
- What are its advantages and challenges?
- How do you maintain and succeed with pump therapy?

What Is an Insulin Pump?

An insulin pump is a small, computerized device programmed to administer small amounts of insulin continuously throughout a 24-hour period. It is comparable in size to a cell phone or pager. Insulin is delivered from the pump through tubing into a small Teflon or steel cannula inserted under the skin. The pump is worn outside the body, carried in a pocket or clipped to a piece of clothing. Pumps allow you to closely mimic the release of insulin that normally takes place in a body without diabetes. However, it is important to recognize that the child wearing the pump (or the supervising adult) tells the pump how much insulin to deliver. Pumps do not have the ability to automatically vary the insulin dose based on blood glucose levels. A pump is only as smart as the person controlling it!

In general, a pump consists of 3 components:

- The pump itself
- A reservoir
- An infusion set

The pump's reservoir, a special type of syringe, is filled with insulin and placed inside the pump. Most current pumps are attached to the body by tubing, which connects the insulin-containing reservoir to an infusion set. The infusion set consists of either a small, flexible, Teflon tube called a cannula or a steel needle. The cannula is inserted under the skin into the fatty tissue with a small needle, either manually or with an insertion device. The needle is then removed, leaving the small Teflon tube just under the skin, which is held in place with tape. This system allows insulin to travel from the reservoir in the pump, into the tubing, through the cannula (or steel needle) of the infusion set, and into the fatty tissue of the body to be absorbed.

Some pumps, called patch pumps, do not have tubing. In these, the insulin-holding device or pod is placed directly on the skin, and functions as the infusion set as well. The pump is controlled by a remote control device the size of a blood glucose meter, and inserts the cannula beneath the skin for you. The amount and rate of insulin infusion is regulated by the pump, which in turn is programmed by the person wearing the pump, or the supervising adult.

Infusion sets can be placed anywhere you would give an injection, as long as there is sufficient fatty tissue. These sites include the:

- Abdomen
- Buttocks
- Hips
- Thighs
- Arms

Infusion set site locations (commonly referred to as *pump sites*) need to be rotated just as you would with injection sites in order to prevent hypertrophy and/or atrophy. It is recommended that the cannula, tubing (if applicable), and insulin in the pump reservoir be changed every 2 days to prevent infection.

How Does Insulin Delivery Work?

Only rapid acting insulin analogs (aspart, glulisine, and lispro) are used in insulin pumps. Since the pump administers small doses of rapid-acting insulin continually throughout the day and night, there is no need for long-acting insulin, as there is with injection therapy. There are 2 basic modes of insulin delivery in insulin pumps: basal and bolus.

Basal Insulin

Basal insulin is background insulin. Its purpose is to keep the blood glucose stable between meals and overnight. It does this by continuously releasing small amounts (1/10 of a unit of insulin, for example), or drips of insulin. Basal rates, or the amounts of insulin released each hour, are programmed into the pump by the pump user, parent, or healthcare provider, and are automatically delivered. Assuming pump malfunction does not occur, the pump will continue to deliver the basal rates as they are programmed until the person wearing the pump tells it to stop or to go at a different rate, or there is no more insulin in the reservoir. Pumps allow for different basal rates to be programmed for different times of day. Depending on the type of insulin pump, you have the capability of programming up to 12, 24, or even 48 different basal rates per day. Most children on pumps are successful using 4 to 6 different rates; but this is highly individualized. You can also adjust basal rates for a short term, known as temporary basal rates, for the duration of particular activities or circumstances, in order to meet your child's individual insulin needs.

Bolus Insulin

Bolus doses are bursts of insulin given in addition to the basal insulin. This method of administration is for your food and correction insulin. Bolus doses are given either before eating, to cover the food you plan to eat, or to correct (bring down) random high blood glucose levels. Most people determine their bolus doses using individualized ratios, referred to as *insulin-to-carbohydrate ratios* and *sensitivity factors* (or *correction factors*). Although the ratios used to calculate the bolus doses can often be programmed into the pump, the actual bolus doses are not preprogrammed and must be manually entered into the pump. Therefore every time a bolus dose needs to be taken, the child wearing the pump (or the supervising adult) must tell the pump how much insulin to deliver.

In order to better match the action of insulin to the absorption of food your child eats, meal boluses, or any bolus taken to cover carbohydrates, should be given at least 10 to 15 minutes before eating. A recent study showed that in children and teens on insulin pump therapy, it takes approximately 90 to 120 minutes after a bolus is given before rapid-acting insulin will have its maximum effect on blood glucose levels. Therefore, if a meal bolus is given during or after a meal, rather than before, it is likely to result in a dramatic spike in the blood glucose level. By giving bolus doses approximately 15 minutes before eating, you can reduce the level of the spike resulting from the meal. Timing of the bolus doses should be individualized. For example, toddlers frequently have to receive their insulin after eating due to their often erratic eating behaviors. Additionally, if the pre-meal blood glucose level is high (in need of a correction bolus), or if your child is more resistant to insulin at that time of day, the bolus should be given even further in advance.

When giving a correction bolus, you must be aware of the risk of overlapping boluses. The duration of insulin action can vary from person to person. Generally, rapid-acting insulin takes 3-5 hours to fully run its course. Always keep in mind the size and timing of the last bolus, and whether or not it may still be acting in your child's body. Using an insulin pump, you have the capability to look back in the bolus history to determine exactly when the last bolus was given. Many pumps also have a safety feature that attempts to calculate how much insulin may still be acting from a previous bolus.

Basal and bolus doses are individually determined. Initially, your child's diabetes healthcare team prescribes these rates. As you and your child become more familiar with the pump, you will work with your diabetes healthcare team to adjust these rates and ratios as needed.

Starting and Maintaining Insulin Pump Therapy

Pump therapy requires a basal/bolus insulin program. Now that you know what these terms mean, you may be wondering how your diabetes care team will determine these individualized doses for your child. It can be helpful to know where these doses come from. They are actually calculated using a somewhat standard equation. **Caution** — when starting pump therapy, wait for your healthcare team to work with you to set your child's basal rates, and bolus ratios.

Total Daily Dose

The first step is to determine the pre-pump total daily dose (TDD) of insulin. This is the total amount of insulin, regardless of the type, given in one day. It is calculated by adding together all rapid- and long-acting insulin doses given throughout an entire day. The body often uses insulin infused by a pump more efficiently than when injected by syringe. Therefore, the total amount of insulin your child needs may decrease when starting pump therapy. Depending on your child's A1C (the reflection of the average glucose control for the past 2-3 months) as well as his or her frequency of hypoglycemia, the diabetes health-care team may use 75-100% of the pre-pump TDD when determining the TDD for the new pump program. If the A1C is high, the provider may choose to be initially aggressive to prevent further hyperglycemia, perhaps using 90-100% of the pre-pump TDD. However, if someone has a lower A1C, or has frequent hypoglycemia, it is wise to start out with a more conservative TDD to prevent hypoglycemia when starting on pump therapy.

Calculating the Basal Rate

In general, a good percentage ratio of basal to bolus insulin is about 50/50. About half of the TDD should be received from basal insulin and the other half from boluses. Once the new TDD is determined, the total is divided in half to get the total basal insulin. This is the amount of basal insulin received over 24 hours. Therefore, if you divide the total basal dose by 24 hours, you have the basal rate per hour. When initially starting pump therapy, the basal rate is usually kept at one constant rate. Throughout the first few weeks (and even months) these rates will most likely be adjusted for different times of day to best meet your child's insulin needs. Frequent blood glucose monitoring is required to determine where adjustments are needed.

Calculating the Insulin to Carbohydrate Ratio

Your child's diabetes care team will use standard equations to initially determine the bolus ratios. The insulin-to-carbohydrate ratio (I:Carb) is the amount of carbohydrates (in grams) that 1 unit of insulin will cover. For example, an insulin-to-carbohydrate ratio of 1:10 means that for every 10 grams of carbohydrate eaten, 1 unit of insulin must be taken. The I:Carb ratio is calculated using the 450 or 500 Rule. This is a rough estimate, and your child's ratio will more than likely change as you and your healthcare team make needed adjustments, but it is a good starting point. The 450 or 500 Rule states that the insulin-to-carbohydrate ratio can be estimated by dividing 450 or 500 by TDD.

Calculating the Sensitivity Factor

Similarly, the sensitivity factor (SF) can be estimated using the 1650 Rule. The sensitivity factor (also called the correction factor) is the number of points (mg/dL) the blood glucose will drop after 1 unit of insulin is given. For example, a SF of 50 means that 1 unit of insulin will bring the blood glucose down 50 points (mg/dL). Using the 1650 Rule, you divide 1650 by the TDD to estimate the sensitivity or correction factor.

Basal rates and bolus ratios are highly individualized. The effectiveness of these doses must be continually assessed, adjusted, and re-assessed. When initially starting on a pump, it takes a lot of extra work not only on the part of your child, but also from the rest of the family. It requires increased blood glucose monitoring throughout the day and night, and careful record keeping. A member of your diabetes care team reviews your logbook and makes adjustments where they are needed. In children and teens with type 1 diabetes, you can expect that these rates and ratios will need to be changed frequently, due to growth and other factors. Once you become more comfortable with the pump and learn how to evaluate the effectiveness of these doses, you may recognize when the doses are not working well, and can work with your diabetes care team to adjust them. Eventually, you may start adjusting things on your own!

Advantages and Challenges of Insulin Pump Therapy

Pump therapy has many advantages over injection therapy. Flexibility, freedom, dosage precision, and improved glucose are just a few. The advantages of pump therapy may be very appealing for your child and for you as parents. However, insulin pump use also comes with challenges and it's extremely important the entire family is aware of, and ready for, these challenges. It is important to identify personal pros and cons of pump therapy for you and your child to help determine if pump therapy might be a good choice.

Table 5-1. Advantages and Challenges of Insulin Pump Therapy (CSII)

Advantages	Challenges
Closest to physiological insulin replacement	Requires more work, not less, than injection therapy
Flexibility and freedom	Catheter site insertion issues and risk of infection
Dosage precision	Risk of hyperglycemia (high blood glucose) and diabetic ketoacidosis (DKA)
Insulin delivery and ability to better match insulin to food, exercise and other factors	Body image
Special features available	Expense
Improved glucose control	Weight gain
Decreased hypoglycemia (low blood glucose)	

Some families considering pump therapy have a pre-misconception that the pump will make life, in regards to diabetes management, much easier. In the long run, this can turn out to be true; but it cannot happen without putting a lot of work into it first. Pump therapy can be compared to taking an advanced level class in school. Simply enrolling your child in the class is not going to guarantee that he or she will excel in it. Excelling in an advanced class requires a lot of hard work, discipline, and support from the child's teacher and family. Comparably, pump therapy requires more work, not less, than multiple daily injections. Pump therapy requires infusion set site changes, frequent blood glucose monitoring, the ability to problem solve, and proficiency in carbohydrate counting. Table 5-1 outlines the advantages and challenges of insulin pump therapy. Each item is discussed in detail below.

Advantages

- **Closest physiological match.** One of the advantages of using an insulin pump is the ability to closely match the normal physiological production and release of insulin. In a person who does not have diabetes, the pancreas releases very precise amounts of insulin. It knows the exact amount needed to cover the carbohydrates being eaten. It knows when to slow down the release, for example when exercise occurs, and it knows when to increase the production and release of insulin, for example when a very large meal is eaten. Although pump therapy is not by any means an exact or perfect science, it helps people with diabetes get one step closer to being able to mimic this complex physiologic function. The challenge is being able to think like a pancreas (and remembering to!).

- **Flexibility.** Another advantage to using a pump is the flexibility it offers in regards to mealtimes, physical activity, sleeping, and family schedules. Different basal rates or temporary basal rates can be programmed for different times of day. This can be helpful in a variety of situations. For example, perhaps your child experiences high blood glucose levels in the early morning. Many children who have diabetes experience this phenomenon (called the dawn phenomenon) due to the release of hormones in early morning hours that counteract the action of insulin, making the body more resistant to insulin. Using an insulin pump, you can set higher basal rates for this time period to accommodate the body's need for more insulin. Conversely, you can also lower basal rates at a particular time of day when your child is prone to have low blood glucose levels; or you could set a temporary rate to adjust for a specific activity. Meal times and sleeping schedules can also be more flexible and less regimented using an insulin pump. Since the pump only uses rapid-acting insulin, it eliminates the need to have a snack or meal at a specific time of day due to a peak in long-acting insulin. This feature also allows kids to sleep late on the weekends, because they don't have to worry about taking an injection in the morning.
- **Precision.** Insulin pumps allow for very precise amounts of insulin to be delivered. Some pumps deliver insulin to the hundredth or even thousandth of a unit (.05 or .025), which would be impossible to measure using a syringe. This can be especially helpful when fine-tuning basal rates, particularly for small children who require very small doses of insulin.
- **Insulin delivery.** Insulin delivery with insulin pumps is also an advantage. The delivery is more predictable, more readily available, and can be individualized to better match food intake and other factors. If your child needs to bolus for a meal or to correct

for a high blood glucose level, the insulin is right there, at the push of a button; there is no need to gather supplies or worry about having everything you need. Furthermore, the infusion sets, after being inserted, are kept in place for 2-3 days, greatly reducing the pain, trauma and perhaps anxiety surrounding the need to give multiple injections each day.

- **Special features.** All the pumps offer a variety of special features. Most pumps currently on the market have been given the name smart pumps. This means the pump has a feature that will calculate a suggested insulin dose using pre-programmed ratios. It calculates the dose based on the current blood glucose level and the amount of carbohydrates you plan to eat. The person wearing the pump must enter a current blood glucose value as well as the number of carbs into the pump. The pump does not have the capability to check your blood glucose level or know how many carbohydrates you are eating. Many pumps also offer an insulin on board feature. When calculating the suggested dose, this safety feature takes into account the amount of insulin you may still have working in your body from a previous bolus. Other special features some pumps may offer include: special bolus programs (dual wave bolus/combination wave bolus, extended/square wave bolus), built in food database programs, the ability to program multiple basal patterns (for example pattern A could be used for school days and pattern B for the weekends), and the option to set reminder alarms.
- **Improved glucose control and reduced hypoglycemia.** For all of these reasons, some people experience better blood glucose control using an insulin pump while potentially reducing the frequency of hypoglycemia. There are many factors that can contribute to hypoglycemia. The peaks of intermediate- and long-acting insulins, which can be unpredictable at times, are a common cause in persons on multiple daily injections. Pump therapy eliminates this factor, which can help reduce (but not eliminate) episodes of hypoglycemia. Whether your child is on injection therapy or insulin pump therapy, hypoglycemia is treated the same. Suspending the pump as a means of treating a low blood

glucose is not effective. When you make a change to the basal rate, or suspend it, you do not see the effects of that change for approximately 1-2 hours. So, suspending your pump in response to a low blood glucose level results in the hypoglycemic event lasting for a longer period of time, followed in a couple of hours by high blood glucose levels.

Challenges

- **Site insertions and risk of infection.** Some find infusion set insertions and site changes to be inconvenient and time consuming. For some children this process is painful and may cause anxiousness. There is also risk of skin irritation or even infection at the insertion site. It is very important to change the sites as recommended, every 2-3 days, and to use clean technique when inserting new infusion sets. You should always wash your hands and clean the site thoroughly before insertion.
- **Pump start process.** The initial start-up when beginning pump therapy takes time, effort and extra blood glucose monitoring. This process can be very challenging for both the child wearing the pump and the family or other caretakers involved.
- **Hyperglycemia and Diabetic Ketoacidosis (DKA).** Pump failure and kinking of the cannula or tubing can result in high blood glucose levels or diabetic ketoacidosis (DKA). As we have discussed, pump therapy generally does not involve the use of long-acting insulin. Therefore, if insulin delivery is cut off or blocked, it will result in high blood glucose levels, which can rapidly progress to a dangerous situation. Persons on insulin pumps are at a higher risk for developing DKA because of these factors. This is one of the reasons pump therapy requires more frequent blood glucose monitoring. Whenever a blood glucose level is greater than 250 mg/dL, the blood or urine should be checked for the presence of ketones. After determining whether or not ketones are present, try to troubleshoot the cause of the high blood glucose level. Check the bolus history to confirm that all meal boluses were delivered; ensure the pump itself is working properly; check the tubing for any

kinks or air bubbles; and look at the actual infusion site and feel for any insulin that may have leaked out (indicating that the cannula may be kinked or coming out). If the cause can be determined, correct the problem (change the site, prime the tubing, etc.) and deliver a correction bolus through the pump. When using the insulin pump to correct a high blood glucose level, it is always important to re-check the blood glucose level in 1 hour to ensure the glucose is coming down. If the blood glucose level has continued to rise, it should be assumed the problem is pump related. In this situation you must check for ketones, administer a correction dose by injection (using a syringe) and change the pump infusion site. If ketones are present (urine ketones or blood ketones of 0.6 mmol/l or greater), you should contact your child's diabetes healthcare team for guidance.

- **Body image.** Another challenge many kids and teens face when wearing a pump has to do with body image. Some don't like the feeling of being attached to something 24 hours a day, or don't want to worry about where to wear their pump on their clothing. This visible and constant reminder of their diabetes may lead to increased questions from friends and/or complete strangers about what the device is, and what it is for. For some people on pumps, particularly children and adolescents, this can be very frustrating, embarrassing, or just simply a bother.
- **Expense.** Pump therapy is more expensive than injection therapy. Most insurance companies cover at least a portion of the cost, but if you do not have adequate health insurance, you need to consider the additional costs associated with the pump before purchasing one.
- **Weight Gain.** Weight gain is often the result of improved glucose control. This will be discussed in more detail later.

Is My Child a Candidate for Pump Therapy?

Determining whether or not to use an insulin pump is a big decision. If you and your child are considering pump therapy, there are many things you should think about before jumping in. Support from the family and a diabetes healthcare team skilled in initiating and supporting ongoing pump education is needed to ensure safety and a positive outcome. One of the first steps when determining whether or not your child would be a good candidate for pump therapy is to talk to your child. Your child is the person who will be wearing the pump all of the time, so it is of extreme importance to make sure he or she is on board with the decision. Experts suggest having your child ask him or herself:

- How will I feel about having a visible sign of my diabetes?
- Where will I wear the pump?
- How will I respond when friends or even strangers ask me what it is?
- How do I feel about being attached to something 24 hours a day?

Make sure that you and/or your child have the skills needed to use the pump. You and/or your child must be able to program the pump. The person wearing the pump, or whoever is administering the bolus doses, must have the ability to count carbohydrates. Problem-solving skills are also needed, because as with any computerized mechanical device, problems are bound to happen.

Timing is an important factor in making the decision to start pump therapy. Determining the appropriate time to start an insulin pump is very important for 2 key reasons: the initiation process requires extra work for everyone involved, and the pump start process often requires frequent clinic visits. Blood glucose levels need to be checked several times throughout the day and night. Many providers have parents keep a log of their child's blood glucose levels, food intake, and exercise; some may even ask for the person wearing the pump to fast for several hours at a time, in order to assess the basal rate settings. Given these demanding requirements, you will want to look at your schedules and give careful thought to when to start on the pump. Pump management needs to begin when the child wearing the pump and the family can focus on the tasks required and on developing new knowledge and skills.

What is involved in starting insulin pump therapy?

Once careful thought has been given to pump therapy, and you have decided to pursue it, the next step is to contact your diabetes healthcare team. Many healthcare providers specializing in diabetes will have pump evaluation and pump-start protocols in place. Ideally, this includes a multidisciplinary team evaluation, intensive education, careful monitoring, and initial assessments, as well as ongoing evaluations.

Expense, as discussed, can be a challenge for some families. One of the first things you should look into when pursuing pump therapy is your insurance coverage. Before going any further in the process, evaluate whether or not pump therapy is financially feasible for your family.

There are a variety of insulin pumps and pump supplies currently available. Each offers a variety of special features and unique characteristics. Choosing a pump is a big decision. The device you, your child, the healthcare team, and perhaps the insurance company (by way of their pump formulary) select will be your child's pump for 4 to 5 years. It is important to discuss what features you are looking for and that you do your homework, determining which pump will best meet your child's needs.

More information on individual insulin pumps is available at the individual pump company's web site. At the time of this printing, the following web sites will provide information:

- Animas Corporation: www.animascorp.com/
- Roche: www.disetronic-usa.com/
- Insulet Corporation: www.myomnipod.com/
- Medtronic Diabetes: www.minimed.com/
- Nipro Diabetes Systems: www.niprodiabetes.com/
- Sooil Development Co. Ltd: www.sooil.com/

The actual process of starting pump therapy requires a lot of education. The first step for pump start programs may be a saline (sterile salt water) start. At this visit, the mechanical and technical aspects of the pump are taught. Your physician prescribes basal rates and bolus ratios and you learn to program them into the pump. You are taught how to insert an infusion set and the pump is loaded with a reservoir containing sterile saline. During this time, your child wears the pump (with insulin or saline in it); if using saline, your child will continue with the current insulin injection therapy.

Starting insulin in the pump is a major step to insulin pump therapy. Prior to this visit, be sure to get instructions from your diabetes healthcare team regarding the dose of insulin to take the night before and/or morning of the insulin start. This phase of pump initiation requires extra blood glucose monitoring. Many providers will ask that you check your child's blood glucose before and after meals, as well as several other times throughout the day and night. Some may even ask the child wearing the pump to fast for a few hours at a time, at different times of day, in order to assess the basal rates. You will also be asked to keep a logbook. Careful record keeping of blood glucoses, food intake and exercise is essential to fine-tuning the basal rates, carbohydrate ratio(s), and sensitivity factor(s).

Frequent follow-up visits and phone calls should be expected when starting a pump for the first time. It is likely your child will start insulin pump therapy with 1 constant basal rate, 1 carbohydrate ratio, and 1 sensitivity factor. Using your logbook and notes, the provider will make adjustments to your child's doses. It is likely the doses will need to be adjusted frequently during the initial start-up period. It can take weeks to months to adjust them to a point where you feel they are working well most of the time; it can take a similar amount of time for you and your child to get to the point of feeling completely comfortable using the pump. However, the extra work and effort in the beginning weeks of pump therapy will pay off in the long run.

Maintaining and Succeeding with Insulin Pump Therapy

Maintaining pump therapy involves a high level of diabetes care. It requires commitment from the parents to provide support and help with daily diabetes management. Regardless of your child's age, parental involvement is very important in managing diabetes and in helping to succeed with pump therapy. Sometimes parents become less involved with diabetes management when their child starts pump therapy. This can happen for several reasons. In many instances, the child may learn how to use and program the pump faster than the parents. This may leave the parents feeling incapable of helping. Additionally, the child may be looking for more independence, and perhaps resisting parental involvement. Experts report that some parents may feel like they are invading the privacy of their child by helping with pump programming because the pump essentially becomes a part of the child's body. Any combination of these things might cause parents to become less involved in the diabetes management of their child, particularly if the parents already feel burned out on diabetes management and need a break. However, it is so important that you as parents stay involved!

Your role as helper and supporter will continually change, but should never become non-existent. When your child first starts on a pump, you may be an active player in his diabetes management, doing nearly everything for him, other than physically wearing the pump. As he gets older, and is ready and able to take on more tasks, your role may change to more of a supportive role. Rather than being an active player, you might function more as a cheerleader. Nevertheless, you must always remain involved. You shouldn't assume that just because your child learns how to do a certain task that he won't need help with it anymore. There may be times when your child has too much on his plate, or is feeling burned out. These are times when you may need to jump back in and help relieve some of that burden. Don't underestimate your value as a member of your child's diabetes care team. Children and teens benefit enormously from positive family involvement with diabetes pump-related tasks.

Planning ahead is particularly important with insulin pump therapy. In addition to carrying a blood glucose meter kit, fast-acting carbohydrates, etc., always carry back-up insulin and syringes or an insulin pen, a spare infusion set and reservoir, and spare batteries. Remember, when using an insulin pump, there isn't any long-acting insulin in the background; if your child's pump malfunctions or breaks, or if the infusion set is pulled out, you need to be prepared. Discuss with your diabetes care team what you and your child need to carry with you, and what you should have on hand at home in case of a pump-related problem. Also, come up with a plan, so you and your child will know exactly what do in the event the pump breaks.

If you are experiencing a pump malfunction, after checking your child's blood glucose level and giving an insulin correction dose (by injection) if needed, you should call the pump company helpline. The number is generally on the back of the pump and the people handling the calls are specially trained to troubleshoot pump-related problems. They may be able to determine the problem and assist you in fixing it over the phone. However, if the pump needs to be replaced or fixed, or if for some reason you are unable to call the helpline right away, you need to be prepared to give your child insulin by syringe or insulin pen. Have vials (or pens) of long-acting and rapid-acting insulin on hand.

Throughout pump therapy, it is important to maintain realistic expectations about what the pump can and cannot do for your child. Although some may see improved glucose control in the first 3 to 6 months after starting a pump, over time, blood glucose levels may return to pre-pump levels. Diabetes control may even worsen over time. Remember, the pump is only as successful as the person controlling it. Used as it is designed to be, the pump can be a great tool; but if you and your child don't know how or don't use is properly, all the technology offered by a pump can be wasted.

Insulin pump therapy is not an exact science. No two persons are exactly the same and because of this everything must be individualized. Keep in mind that there are many factors that influence blood glucose levels — hormones, activity level, food, and stresses arc just a few. These factors may change on a monthly, weekly, or even daily basis — particularly in growing children. Because of this, you and your child must work with your diabetes care team to evaluate what is working, and what needs to be changed.

Preventing Weight Gain

Some people who start insulin pump therapy may gain weight initially, as their blood glucose control improves. When blood glucose levels are high, the body is unable to use the glucose for energy; but when the glucose is used rather than being flushed out in the urine, it can lead to weight gain. Working with a Registered Dietitian before and throughout pump therapy can help to prevent this from occurring.

Some individuals starting pump therapy may gain weight for a different reason. With the newfound flexibility and freedom of being able to eat whenever they want at the push of a button, some may find themselves eating more throughout the day, which can lead to weight gain. Simply because insulin is easier to deliver with a pump, it does not mean you and your child can throw healthy eating out the window. Children and teens need to be taught the importance of healthy eating habits, moderation, and exercise whether they are on an insulin pump or multiple daily injections . . . Or for that matter, regardless of whether or not they have diabetes at all.

Pump Vacation

At some point, there will probably come a time when your child wants to come off of the pump. This may be for a short time — for example, if you are taking a family vacation to the beach — or for a longer period if he or she is burned out from wearing the pump. Before your child takes a pump vacation, it is important to discuss these plans with your diabetes healthcare team. You'll review your back-up insulin plan with your provider and discuss other possible insulin therapy options.

In order to unhook for longer than 90-120 minutes, some utilize a form of un-tethered pumping, using backup long-acting insulin, either glargine (Lantus) or detemir (Levemir). Using this program, you take a percentage of your normal total basal dose through an injection of long-acting insulin. The remaining basal dose is administered by the insulin pump (each of the original hourly basal rates would be reduced to account for the percentage of long-acting insulin given). This allows more flexibility when it comes to disconnecting from the pump, since the long-acting insulin provides background insulin that lasts through the day.

Advanced Pumping

Once you have the basics of the standard basal and bolus down, you may want to experiment with some of the more advanced tools your pump offers. Keep in mind that each time you change a setting, or try something new, you and your child will be performing an experiment. After each experiment you will gather information and take what you learned to make the necessary adjustments. Often, the experiment will need to be repeated multiple times. It takes trial and error, frequent blood glucose monitoring, and careful note taking to get things to work right most of the time (it will never work right all of the time).

Many pumps offer special insulin delivery programs. Temporary basal rates can be helpful in the prevention of hypoglycemia related to exercise. Temporary rates can also be used when managing times of increased insulin needs, such as sick days.

Special bolus programs, such as a dual/combination wave or extended/ square wave, are also available in most pumps. These different types of boluses offer some variety in how a meal bolus is delivered. This can be helpful when taking insulin for meals that are very high in fat and/or protein, or perhaps to cover foods that will be eaten over a long period of time (for example, a 5 course meal).

- **A dual or combination wave bolus** releases 2 bursts of insulin. The first burst — a percentage of the total bolus, which you choose — is delivered initially, just as a normal bolus would be delivered. The second delivery (the remaining amount of the total dose), however, is spread out over an amount of time that you choose. A good starting point when bolusing for a meal with high fat content, like pizza, is to deliver 50% initially, and the remaining 50% over 2-3 hours. The first few times performing this experiment it is important to check your blood glucose often, to determine if adjustments need to be made. You may find, for example, that your blood glucose is high 2 hours after eating, in which case you may need more insulin (perhaps 60% of the total bolus) initially. You may also find that the second wave's length of duration may need to be longer or shorter.

- **An extended or square wave bolus** takes the entire bolus and delivers it over a duration of time that you determine. This program can be very helpful when dealing with situations where there is delayed gastric absorption and emptying. This could be the result of eating a food that has a low glycemic index or perhaps the result of a condition called gastroparesis. Some also find this type of bolus useful when they anticipate eating over a long period of time (*e.g.*, a 5 course meal).

Remember, this is not an exact science. What works for one person on a pump may not necessarily work for you or your child. Furthermore, what works for your child at one point in time, may not work a few weeks or months later! This is just one of the many challenging aspects of managing diabetes in children; their bodies, insulin needs, and responses to various factors which influence blood glucose levels are constantly changing.

Worsening Control and How to Improve the Situation

After your child has been on the pump for a while, and everyone is more comfortable with it, you may find that you and your child become somewhat lax with performing certain pump-related tasks: checking blood glucose levels less frequently, forgetting to bolus, becoming careless with carbohydrate counting, or disconnecting the pump for extended periods of time without any backup or replacement insulin. Any combination of these things can lead to deterioration in diabetes control. An overall decrease in the amount of family involvement can be a factor as well.

In order to improve the situation, it is essential that you as parents are involved enough in your child's care to recognize the problem, and to help provide a solution. Often just increasing family involvement and support will help improve glucose control. Be aware of signs of diabetes burnout in your child, and be prepared to jump in and help whenever they need you. Talk with your healthcare team and discuss what you and your child are struggling with. Only if they are aware of the problem can they help you to problem-solve and offer suggestions.

If the cause of worsening control seems to be that you and your child are just not paying as close attention to pump-related tasks as you once did, often returning (even for a week or two) to the initial pump-start routine — in relation to checking blood glucose levels frequently, keeping a handwritten logbook, weighing and measuring foods, and perhaps working with a Registered Dietitian to get a refresher course on carbohydrate counting — can be very beneficial.

When to Consider Switching Back to Insulin Injections

Insulin pump therapy is not for everyone. Some may try the pump and make a personal decision that the benefits do not outweigh the drawbacks. Some people struggling with their diabetes management on pump therapy may make a permanent transition back to injections. The main reasons for terminating pump therapy include burnout, worsening blood glucose control, infusion site problems, weight gain, or body image concerns. Discuss different insulin therapy options with your healthcare team, and together, come up with a realistic plan for improving diabetes management. Regardless of the reason for going off the pump, it is important to remain supportive of your child, and to avoid any feelings of shame, guilt, or failure on the part of you or your child.

Summary

Insulin pump therapy uses an exciting piece of technology; however, it is not for everyone. It has advantages and disadvantages. Regardless of whether your family is considering pump therapy, starting pump therapy, maintaining pump therapy, or perhaps even burned out on pump therapy, it is essential to keep the lines of communication open between the child wearing the pump, the parents and the diabetes healthcare team. Remember that insulin pump therapy, just like diabetes management in general, is a team effort.

References and Resources

Butler, D. To pump, or not to pump? *Diabetes Self Management*. 2005; 22(5):74-80.

Swan KL, Weinzimer ST. Effect of puberty on the pharmacodynamic and pharmacokinetic properties of insulin pump therapy in youth with type 1 diabetes. *Diabetes Care*. 2008; 31:44-46.

Wolpert H. You don't need a sermon; The pump advantage; Laying the foundation; Getting your basal rates on track, In: *Smart Pumping for People with Diabetes*. Alexandria, VA: American Diabetes Association; 2002:2-39.

Chase PH, Owen S, Gaston J, Block J. Insulin pumps. In: *Understanding Diabetes*, 11th edition. Denver, CO: Children's Diabetes Foundation; 2006:279-298.

Edelman S. The "un-tethered" regimen. Children with Diabetes Website. 2005. Available at: http://www.childrenwithdiabetes.com/clinic/untethered.htm. Accessed April 5, 2009.

Web sites:

- www.diabetesnet.com
- www.childrenwithdiabetes.com
- www.insulin-pumpers.org
- www.childrenwithdiabetes.com
- Animas Corporation: www.animascorp.com
- Roche: www.disetronic-usa.com
- Insulet Corporation: www.myomnipod.com
- Medtronic Diabetes: www.minimed.com
- Nipro Diabetes Systems: www.niprodiabetes.com
- Sooil Development Co. Ltd: www.sooil.com

6

Monitoring Glucose and Ketones

Monitoring is one of the cornerstones of diabetes management. Without the information obtained from monitoring, you and your healthcare team cannot make the best choices on how to manage your child's diabetes. The information obtained from the different types of monitoring that will be discussed in this chapter gives you the pieces to a puzzle. The more pieces of the puzzle that you have, the clearer the picture will be. You will be able to use this information:

- To make adjustments for both well and sick days.
- To understand whether or not the treatment approaches are working.
- For exercise management, interpretation of behavior, driving safety, and distinction between symptoms of high or low blood glucose.
- To determine the right choices for your child.

You will, undoubtedly, be more confident in the treatment decisions that you make.

In this section we will discuss 4 types of monitoring:

- Blood Glucose Monitoring (BGM)
- Ketone Monitoring
  - Blood Ketone Monitoring
  - Urine Ketone Monitoring
- Hemoglobin A1C (A1C) and Estimated Average Glucose (eAG)
- Continuous Glucose Monitoring (CGM)

Blood Glucose Monitoring

History

Blood glucose meters for home use became available in 1969 and more commonplace in the 1980s. Prior to this, diabetes was managed by checking urine for glucose. This is not the most accurate method, though, as the glucose in urine reflects what the blood glucose was at least 2-3 hours ago. Checking for glucose in urine does not allow for informed real-time treatment decisions. The first blood glucose meters heralded a breakthrough in diabetes care but left much room for improvement. They were large in size, had long testing times, and were prone to errors in user technique. Today, meters are smaller, faster, require smaller amounts of blood and, thus, make the process of checking blood glucose more efficient and tolerable. In 5 seconds or less, a meter can measure the blood glucose and display the result. With this information, you can better manage diabetes because you can treat low blood glucoses and react to high blood glucoses right away. This technology has made remarkable changes in the way we care for diabetes.

Blood Glucose Lingo

How you talk about blood glucose levels and how you react to them is very important. Your response to a particular blood glucose level, as well as the language you use in relation to the number, will help to determine whether or not you will encourage an open dialogue about blood glucose with your child. The following three tips are suggestions to help you with the discussion of monitoring and interpreting blood glucose results.

- **Tip 1:** It is important for all caregivers to use the words blood glucose *CHECK*, not the words blood glucose *TEST*. Your child does not pass or fail a blood glucose check. Your child does not get an A or C or F for the day. The current blood glucose level is simply a number that you use to make a decision in the care of your child regardless of what the number is, whether it is 89 or 152 or 322. Would you want to take a test 4 or more times each day? If you have been calling it a blood glucose test, it is important to try to make a fresh start and call it a blood glucose check. No one can fail. It is a great accomplishment anytime blood glucose is checked. Without this, you won't have the information you need. When you have this information, everyone wins!

- **Tip 2:** Try to use words like *in range* or *out of range* or simply *high* or *low* instead of *good* or *bad* to describe blood glucose levels. A multitude of factors, some of which are in your or your child's control and others that are not, will influence a blood glucose level at any given point in time. Extra carbohydrate or stress may raise the blood glucose but this does not make it bad. Unplanned activity or decreased carbohydrate intake may lower blood glucose but this does not make it "good." Don't judge the number, use the information to problem-solve.
- **Tip 3:** Try not to become too emotional about blood glucose numbers. It is very common at times to feel fear, anger, or frustration when you see high or low blood glucose. Remember these feelings are normal and it is sometimes difficult to not feel this way. It is of utmost importance to never punish your child because of a blood glucose reading. Scolding or accusing your child of cheating or sneaking because of high blood glucose does not solve any diabetes management problems. In fact, it only encourages children to not share information about their diabetes for fear of punishment. What will help is redirecting the energy at problem solving like encouraging extra activity to decrease a high blood glucose. At times, you may need to just let go of an unexplained high or low blood glucose. Sometimes, despite doing everything right, you may not see the results that you want. You must remember there is no such thing as *perfect* blood glucose.

Why You Need to Monitor Blood Glucose

Checking your child's blood glucose will help you and your healthcare team make informed choices about your child's diabetes treatment. Better decisions about food, insulin doses, and activity can be made both immediately and retrospectively. There are important safety reasons for monitoring. Some individuals, especially young children, cannot always recognize the symptoms of low blood glucose. Thus, it helps to decrease the likelihood of a severe low blood glucose. Symptoms of low and high blood glucose can be confused. Even a rapid drop in blood glucose from high to in range can cause the symptoms of a low blood glucose. Thus, the finger-stick lets you confirm what is going on, providing timely information. The information you get from blood glucose checks helps you and your child learn to identify how your child feels within certain ranges of blood glucose. A child who says "my legs don't work," "my words are fuzzy," or who acts sleepy or cranky when the meter reads less than 80 is communicating the best way he or she knows how to ask for help to treat a low blood glucose. You as a parent can begin to recognize these behaviors as symptoms of low blood glucose. You can teach your child how to ask for help when he or she feels these symptoms. The age at which children can recognize their symptoms of low blood glucose varies but is usually between the ages of 5 and 8. However, even an older child is not always able to recognize when a blood glucose is low or high. Monitoring helps you to distinguish if symptoms being felt are truly the result of a low blood glucose or for some other reason.

Most importantly, monitoring helps you to improve your child's overall blood glucose control. Studies have shown that increased frequency of self-monitoring of blood glucose helps in the reduction of hemoglobin A1C, which reduces the risk of long-term complications.

Frequency of Blood Glucose Checks

Your child should have a blood glucose check a minimum of 4 times per day. This includes before breakfast, before lunch, before dinner, and at bedtime. The bedtime check is especially important if your child has been very active that day. The bedtime check will tell you if your child needs extra food to minimize the chances of low blood glucose in the middle of the night. Additional checks should always be done when either high or low blood glucose is suspected. This will allow for appropriate treatment measures to be taken if needed. You may also be asked to sometimes check blood glucose 2 hours after meals to see how well rapid-acting insulin is covering a meal. During times of illness, you may need to check the blood glucose every 2-3 hours including through the night. Your health-care team will help you determine the optimal frequency of monitoring.

Blood Glucose Targets

The goals for blood glucose levels depend on your child's age and the time of day. Table 6-1 outlines the blood glucose levels guidelines recommended by the American Diabetes Association.

Table 6-1. ADA Recommended Blood Glucose Levels

Age	Before Meals	Bedtime/Overnight
Toddlers and Preschoolers (0–6)	100–180 mg/dL	110–200 mg/dL
School age (6–12)	90–180 mg/dL	100–180 mg/dL
Adolescents and Young adults (13–19)	90–130 mg/dL	90–150 mg/dl

How to Check Blood Glucose

BGM is performed using a blood glucose meter. Meters come in different shapes, colors, and sizes and with different features. Preferred features include the need for a small drop of blood, compact size, short monitoring time, a memory system, downloading capability, and accuracy. Many insurance companies have preferred meter brands (meters and strips) for which they provide coverage. You should check with your insurance company to see what will be covered. Test strips are expensive and not reusable so it is important to use a brand that will be covered by your health insurance to minimize expenses. Your healthcare team can help choose which meter best fits the needs of you and your child.

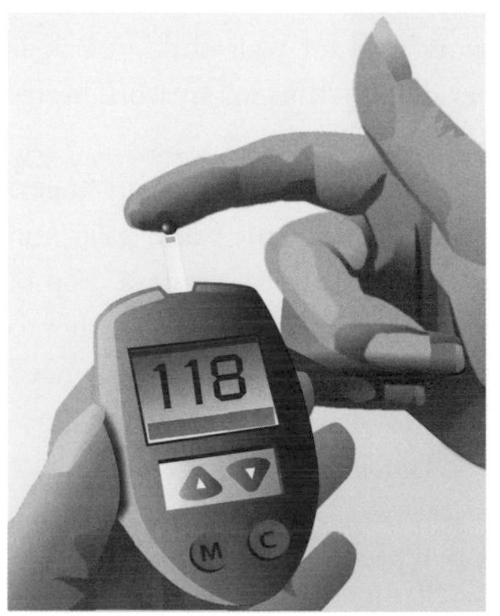

It is important when you get a new meter to go through the basic set-up and set the meter's time and date. This allows you and your healthcare team to obtain accurate information when either the meter memory is reviewed or the meter is downloaded. Most meters require coding. The code is specific to a particular lot of strips. The strip is the part to which blood is applied. Strips come in vials, foil wrapped packages or drums. Strips have expiration dates. It is important to note that strips contained in vials are good for 3 months once opened, even if the expiration date has not been reached. Strips should not be exposed to extremes of temperature. For accurate results, you must use unexpired strips as well as the proper code. Some meters require manual change of the code while others have a code strip or chip. A few meters do not require coding. Read the owner's manual carefully to learn how to use your meter and ask your healthcare team to demonstrate appropriate use of the meter.

To obtain a drop of blood, a lancet and lancing device are used. Your meter will come with these. Lancets are plastic tools, approximately 1 inch in length, with a needle tip on the end. The needle comes in different sizes (gauges). The gauge of the lancet should be as high as possible as a higher gauge means the needle is smaller, causing less discomfort. A gauge of 33 is the finest currently available. You should change the lancet each time a finger-stick is done. This reduces the risk of infection and prevents dulling of the lancet. A dull lancet increases the discomfort as well as makes it difficult to get an adequate drop of blood. It is also important to rotate the fingers used to minimize the formation of calluses. The lancing device is the piece of equipment that holds the lancet. It has a spring-like mechanism that releases the needle towards the fingertip. This helps control how far the needle enters the finger. There are a number of different lancing devices. If the lancing device that comes with the meter does not work well for your child, ask your healthcare team for suggestions of other devices that might work better for him or her.

If you will be using fingertips, you should always ensure clean fingers before checking blood glucose. It is best to wash with warm soap and water. This increases blood flow and makes it easier to obtain a drop of blood. If you have trouble bleeding, you can also rub the hands together to warm them up or shake them below the level of the heart. You may need to milk the finger to get a good drop. Alcohol can also be used but tends to dry out the skin. Whichever method you choose, you need to make sure the hands are dry before doing a finger-stick.

When blood glucose meters were the new technology, only fingers were used for blood glucose checks. Some meters now have alternate site testing capability. Depending on the specific meter, the areas you can use are the forearm, upper arm, palm, thigh, and calf. The main advantage is to possibly decrease the pain associated with blood glucose monitoring and hopefully increase the frequency of blood glucose checks. A different cap is used on the lancing device if you use one of these alternate sites. You may need to rub the area to get good blood flow prior to doing a stick.

If you do use an alternate site, it is important to know that the blood glucose reading is only reliable when blood glucose is not changing quickly. A delay of as much as 20 minutes can occur with the level in alternate sites versus the fingertip when there is a rapid change. Because of this, alternate site testing is not recommended for young children and for anyone else who is not able to recognize symptoms of low blood glucose. Even if you are able to recognize low blood glucose, the recommendation is to do a fingers-tick if a low blood glucose is suspected.

Recording Blood Glucose Results

So now that you have all this information, what do you do with it? For highs or lows, you can make the most appropriate treatment decision immediately. For example, it lets you know what insulin dose to give, whether or not to give a snack before activity, or if a correction dose is needed. But how do you know if overall changes need to be made to prevent highs and lows and keep blood glucose in the target range? To make the most of this information, *record keeping* is *key*. Record keeping allows you to look for patterns as well as to see the impact of a soccer game, a meal and a test at school or an insulin dose. Each meter comes with a logbook but you may find it helpful to make a log that fits your individual needs. Information in the logbook should include date, time, blood glucose level, insulin dose, ketone checks, unusual happenings, such as illness or a party, and any other information that would help your healthcare team and you in making decisions about your child's diabetes management plan.

Many meters have expanded memories and electronic logbooks that can be downloaded. Some blood glucose meters and insulin pumps allow you to enter into them events such as insulin dose, food, and activity. While it is great that meters have this capability, it is still important to try to keep a paper log or at least a notebook allowing you to record unusual occurrences so that you may refer back to the information to help explain highs or lows. Most families will not remember what happened last week when their healthcare provider asks them to identify a possible cause for a high or low. Many families find keeping a logbook to be one of the more challenging tasks of the diabetes plan, but it is crucial. Thus, it is important to find a method that suits your needs as well as your available time. An added benefit of record keeping is the ability it provides you, if you are comfortable, to make changes on your own in between medical appointments.

Ketone Monitoring

Ketones

Ketones are a by-product produced by the human body when stored fat is burned for energy. This will happen when glucose is not available due to insulin deficiency or when the body is in a fasting state. Ketone levels that become too high are very dangerous and can lead to diabetic ketoacidosis (DKA). It is important to note that DKA comes with warning signs which include consistently high blood glucose levels as well as positive ketones in the blood and urine. For a child treated with injection therapy, DKA takes at least 12-24 hours to develop; however, for children treated with insulin pumps, this may occur within 4-5 hours. Given the seriousness of DKA, it is important to remember that ketone monitoring is just as important as blood glucose monitoring, especially during times of illness or stress. It is crucial that you follow your healthcare team's guidelines for when and how to check for ketones and what treatment to follow if ketones are present.

When to Check for Ketones

There are several circumstances that warrant checking for ketones:

- Injected insulin: when the blood glucose (BG) is greater than 250 mg/dL two times in a row. Insulin pump: when BG is greater than 250 mg/dL.
- During times of illness such as a cold, the flu, or a stomach bug.
- When your child complains of stomach pain, nausea or vomit-

ing. (This is especially important because these complaints can actually be signs of having ketones in the blood.)

How to Check for Ketones

Ketones can be monitored both in the blood and the urine. Blood is the preferred method to check although many people still check in the urine. Checking urine has limitations. Just like checking urine for glucose, checking urine for ketones does not reflect the current situation. As mentioned before, this is because urine reflects what happened at least 2-3 hours ago. Also, if urine strips in vials are not stored in the appropriate condition, or are used more than 6 months after first opening the vial, the strips lose accuracy. Moreover, urine strips must be timed exactly. Timing is dependent on the brand of strips used. Another complicating factor is that a person with eyesight problems may have problems interpreting the color variations on the strips. Additionally, it is often difficult to get a sample of urine from young children.

Just as with blood glucose monitoring, blood ketone monitoring lets you know what is going on at that exact moment in time. Ketones appear in the blood first before being removed by the kidneys into the urine. By checking for blood ketones you catch the problem earlier. There is one meter called the Precision Xtra that checks for blood ketones. Though it is better to check for ketones in the blood, if blood ketone strips are not covered by health insurance, you may choose to continue to check ketones in the urine.

Normal Ketone Levels

If using urine strips, ketone levels will be referred to as:

- negative
- trace
- small
- moderate
- large

Other brands will equate each word to a numeric value, for example ranging from 0 to 160 mg/dL. Negative and trace ketone levels do not require intervention. However, any level small or greater will require treatment.

If measuring blood ketones, a numeric value is used:

- Anything less than 0.6 mmdl/L is considered normal.
- Anything greater than or equal to 0.6 mmdl/L requires intervention.
- The following provides guidance on how to interpret the result from measuring blood ketones:

Below 0.6 mmdl/L	Readings below 0.6 mmdl/L are in the normal range.
0.6 to 1.5 mmdl/L	Readings between 0.6 and 1.5 mmdl/L may indicate the development of a problem that may require medical assistance. Patient should follow healthcare provider's instructions.
Above 1.5 mmdl/L	Readings above 1.5 mmdl/L indicate a risk of developing diabetic ketoacidosis (DKA). Patient should contact a healthcare provider immediately for advice.

You should follow the advice of both your healthcare team and the blood ketone strips product insert.

What to Do If Your Child Has Ketones

If more than trace (urine) or greater than 0.6 level (blood) ketones are present, it is important to call your healthcare team for further advice. The only way to get rid of high blood glucose with ketones is to give extra rapid-acting or short-acting insulin as well as increase intake of sugar-free fluids. Fluids help to flush the ketones out of the body. Your healthcare team will help you decide on how much additional insulin to give. You will also need to continue to check your child's blood glucose and ketones every 2-3 hours until there are no ketones in the blood or urine. For additional information, refer to sick day rules in Chapter 11: Sick Days and DKA Prevention.

What is a glycosolated hemoglobin A1C?

The third type of monitoring is the glycosolated hemoglobin A1C, or A1C for short. Just like blood glucose meters, the A1C test has helped in

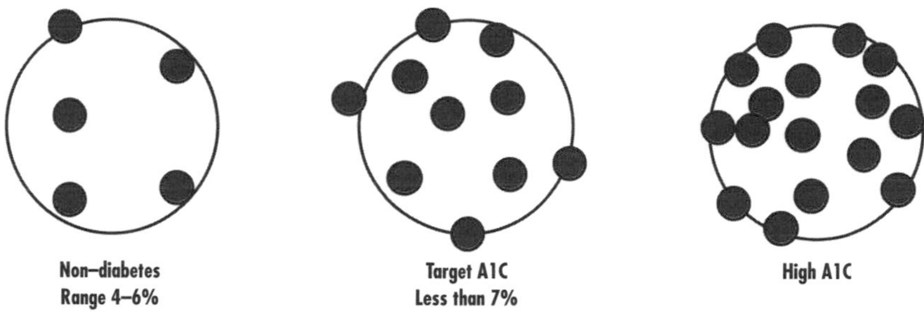

FIGURE 6-1. Graphic Depiction of Glucose Attaching to Hemoglobin at Variable A1C Values

the management of diabetes since the early 1980s. The test measures the amount of glucose that attaches to hemoglobin, part of our red blood cells. As the hemoglobin travels through the bloodstream, it picks up glucose; the more glucose in your blood, the more glucose attaches to the hemoglobin. A good way to think of an A1C is that it is blood glucose with a memory. There is a protein in red blood cells called hemoglobin. It is what carries oxygen to your cells from your lungs. But, in addition to oxygen, glucose also attaches to hemoglobin. This process occurs for all people, whether they have diabetes or not. For people without diabetes, there are standard levels of how much glucose will attach to the hemoglobin (4-6%). For people with diabetes, however, the higher the blood glucose levels have been, the more glucose sticks to the red blood cells. Red blood cells live 2-3 months and the A1C provides the big picture of what has been happening with overall blood glucose during those 2-3 months. It is, however, the past 4-6 weeks that most influence the A1C value. Sometimes it is helpful to think of the A1C as an average blood glucose over a long period.

Table 6-2 shows A1C goals based on age.

Table 6-2. Age-Based A1C Goals

Age (years)	A1C
Toddlers and Preschoolers (0–6)	less than 8.5%
School age (6–12)	less than 6 – 8.0%
Adolescents and Young adults (13–19)	less than 7.5%

Calculating the A1C

The A1C test is done in the clinic, health provider's office, or at a lab. This test should be done every 3 months. It may require that blood be drawn from a vein but many labs can do this test from a finger-stick, making the procedure much more comfortable for your child. It is very similar to the finger-stick used for daily monitoring of blood glucose. What makes this test even more useful is that it can now be done as a Point of Care A1C. This simply means that a result can be obtained in 6-8 minutes, depending on what system is being used. Thus, your healthcare team can have the information available during your visit to make better suggestions for any changes that may be necessary in the diabetes treatment plan.

A1C and Estimated Average Glucose (eAG)

An estimated Average Glucose (eAG) is a new way to present an A1C value in numbers like you see on your child's blood glucose meter. The American Diabetes Association has an eAG calculator available at: http://www.diabetes.org/eag.jsp. Table 6-3 shows how an A1C will be translated from a percentage to a blood glucose value – the eAG.

Continuous Glucose Monitoring

What is it?

Until recently, the only way to monitor blood glucose was with a blood glucose meter. This information is incredibly useful but only provides snapshots of information. A newer tool, known as continuous glucose monitoring (CGM), provides a more complete picture of what is happening to the blood glucose throughout the day and night. It is important to note that CGM does not replace blood glucose checks with a meter; it supplements this information giving you a better understanding of what is happening to glucose levels.

The first generation of continuous glucose monitoring devices was used for retrospective review. The devices recorded and stored glucose data which was later downloaded by your healthcare provider. The newer systems let you see real time glucose data on a screen while you are wearing the device. The device displays a current glucose level and shows you if your glucose is steady or trending up or down.

Table 6-3. A1C Values Expressed as Estimated Average Glucose Values

Average glucose = (28.7 x A1C) – 46.7

A1C (%)	Average Glucose (mg/dL)	A1C (%)	Average Glucose (mg/dL)	A1C (%)	Average Glucose (mg/dL)	A1C (%)	Average Glucose (mg/dL)
5.0	97	8.0	183	11.0	269	14.0	355
5.1	100	8.1	186	11.1	272	14.1	358
5.2	103	8.2	189	11.2	275	14.2	361
5.3	105	8.3	192	11.3	278	14.3	364
5.4	108	8.4	194	11.4	280	14.4	367
5.5	111	8.5	197	11.5	283	14.5	369
5.6	114	8.6	200	11.6	286	14.6	372
5.7	117	8.7	203	11.7	289	14.7	375
5.8	120	8.8	206	11.8	292	14.8	378
5.9	123	8.9	209	11.9	295	14.9	381
6.0	126	9.0	212	12.0	298	15.0	384
6.1	128	9.1	214	12.1	301	15.1	387
6.2	131	9.2	217	12.2	303	15.2	390
6.3	134	9.3	220	12.3	306	15.3	392
6.4	137	9.4	223	12.4	309	15.4	395
6.5	140	9.5	226	12.5	312	15.5	398
6.6	143	9.6	229	12.6	315	15.6	401
6.7	146	9.7	232	12.7	318	15.7	404
6.8	148	9.8	235	12.8	321	15.8	407
6.9	151	9.9	237	12.9	324	15.9	410
7.0	154	10.0	240	13.0	326	16.0	413
7.1	157	10.1	243	13.1	329		
7.2	160	10.2	246	13.2	332		
7.3	163	10.3	249	13.3	335		
7.4	166	10.4	252	13.4	338		
7.5	169	10.5	255	13.5	341		
7.6	171	10.6	258	13.6	344		
7.7	174	10.7	260	13.7	346		
7.8	177	10.8	263	13.8	349		
7.9	180	10.9	266	13.9	352		

Components of CGM Systems

There are 3 components to every CGM system:

- **Sensor.** The sensor is a tiny, flexible electrode that sits underneath the skin in the interstitial fluid. Interstitial fluid is the liquid that surrounds your cells. The sensor is introduced under the skin with a needle and special insertion device that is unique to the brand of CGM being worn. Once inserted, the needle is removed and the sensor is left under the skin and should not be felt. The sensor is worn for 3 to 7 days depending on the brand of CGM.
- **Transmitter.** The transmitter attaches to the sensor and is worn on the body. The transmitter is made of plastic and is waterproof so it can be worn while bathing or swimming. The transmitter is a tiny computer that sends information from the sensor to the receiver wirelessly. You must be within approximately 6 feet of the receiver for the transmitter to send the information, but the exact distance will vary depending on brand of CGM.
- **Receiver.** The receiver displays and stores the glucose information. It is about the size of a pager or an insulin pump. It can be worn on a belt, kept in a pocket or carried in a purse or backpack. It displays a glucose value in real time every 1 to 5 minutes depending on brand of CGM. In addition to the current value, you can see a trend graph that allows you to see

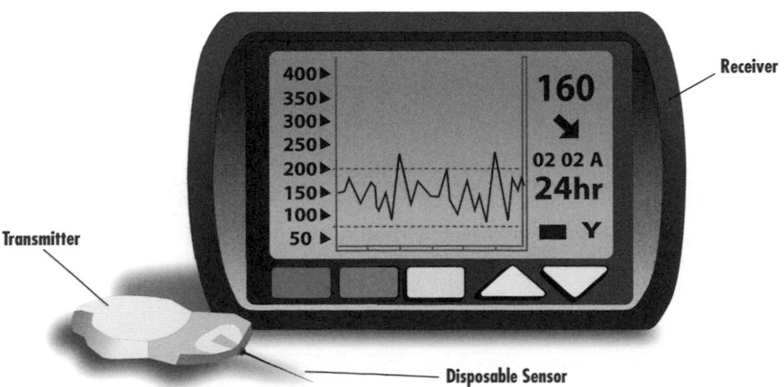

what has happened to the blood glucose over the past 3 to 24 hours. Some devices have arrows that will show if the glucose is rising or falling at a certain rate. The trend information can be used to help guide your treatment decisions.

How CGM Works

The tip of the sensor has an enzyme that breaks down glucose and generates a small electric current that changes depending on your glucose level. This current is converted to a glucose value by calibrating the device with finger-stick blood glucose checks. This is done 1-4 times per day depending on the brand of device. The transmitter sends glucose information to the receiver by radio frequency. All the available products require a warm-up period lasting several hours before the sensor can start. After the warm-up period, a calibration (finger-stick blood glucose) is required. Calibration is key to the accuracy of the CGM device.

The following are tips to help you with the calibration process:

- Do not calibrate the CGM when your glucose is changing rapidly — the best times to do this are before meals and at bedtime and at least 3 hours after food intake and/or insulin dose. Do not calibrate when arrows are present or when the sensor graph display shows a change in glucose level of more than 60 mg/dL over 1 hour.
- Make sure you use clean finger tips when checking blood glucose
- Make sure the glucose meter is coded correctly
- Enter the finger-stick glucose reading immediately

Remember to follow the manufacturer's guidelines for calibrating as well as the recommendations of your healthcare team.

Why Fingerstick Readings Do Not Always Match the Sensor Reading

It is important to know that sensor readings will not be exactly the same as blood glucose readings using your meter. The sensor measures the amount of glucose in your interstitial fluid, while a blood glucose meter measures the glucose in your blood. It is normal to see as much as a 20% difference between the two. It can be even greater if the glucose is changing quickly.

The glucose from your meals is first absorbed into the blood and then passes into the interstitial space before it goes into the cell. It may take as long as 30 minutes for glucose to move from the blood to the interstitial space. This is known as *lag time*.

It is important to keep lag time in mind when interpreting the readings that you are seeing on your receiver. For example, if you eat a meal, the higher glucose number will show first in your blood. Thus, your finger-stick will not match the sensor reading. The senor may report a glucose of 150 while the finger stick shows a reading of 180. This does not mean the sensor is malfunctioning; it is normal physiology. This situation may also occur when the blood glucose is falling rapidly. If a low blood glucose is occurring, the meter may show a level of 70 while the CGM device shows an interstitial glucose of 100. Thus, all treatment decisions need to be made based on finger-stick blood glucose readings.

Available Devices

There are currently 4 FDA-approved devices for use in adults 18 years and older. Two of these devices have pediatric versions that are approved down to the age of 7: the MiniMed Paradigm Real-Time System and the MiniMed Guardian Real-Time System, K versions.

- DexCom's Seven Plus continuous glucose monitoring system determines glucose levels every 30 seconds and transmits glucose information to the receiver every 5 minutes. The sensor is worn for up to 7 days. The receiver can show a 1-, 3-, 6-, 12-, and 24-hour trend graphs. The system has programmable high and low glucose alerts. These alarms can be adjusted and turned on or off. However, as a safety feature, there is a default low glucose alarm of 55 that cannot be turned off. There is an initial 2-hour warm-up period and calibrations are required every 12 hours.
- Medtronic offers 2 systems. One is linked to an insulin pump and the other is a stand-alone device. The MiniMed Paradigm Real-Time System communicates with the Paradigm 522/722 insulin pumps. The MiniMed Guardian Real-Time System communicates with a separate monitor. Both systems transmit

glucose information every 5 minutes for up to 72 hours. High and low glucose alarms can be set according to your needs. A blood glucose calibration is needed 2 hours after insertion, within 6 hours of the initial calibration and then every 12 hours. The Guardian Real-Time System will alarm when the sensor predicts low or high interstitial glucose based on the latest sensor glucose and rate of change. It will also alarm for a rapid rate of change in glucose. Both systems display trend information with direction and rate of change. The Paradigm Real-Time System shows 3- and 24- hour graphs while the Guardian Real-Time System has additional 6- and 12-hour graphs.

- Abbott Diabetes Care's Freestyle Navigator is a 5-day real-time continuous glucose monitor. The Navigator displays blood glucose values every minute with direction and rate of change as well. Blood glucose information can be displayed in 2-, 4-, 6-, 12-, and 24-hour graphs. The system is calibrated 10, 12, 24, and 72 hours after insertion. After the 72-hour mark, no further calibration is needed. The Navigator has predictive alerts for highs and lows that will alarm up to 30 minutes before the time it predicts the low or high blood glucose.

CGM Pros and Cons

There are both advantages and disadvantages to CGM. CGM is not the right choice for everyone. It is important to discuss CGM with your healthcare team to determine the best choice for you.

Pros:

- May reduce the number of finger-sticks needed throughout the day.
- Provides trend information to modify treatment decisions for insulin doses and food intake.
- Helps you learn how certain activities, foods, or stress may affect your glucose.
- Helps to detect post-meal blood glucose spikes.
- May help to prevent or reduce the number of lows.
- May reduce your worry about low and high blood glucose.

- Gives more information to help see what is going on behind the scenes.

Cons:

- May increase the number of fingersticks.
- Adds extra time to daily diabetes management.
- Potential nuisance alarms that may disrupt sleep or classroom activities.
- Possibility of skin irritation, rashes, or infection.
- May cause you to focus too much on your child's diabetes.
- CGM information may be too overwhelming, confusing, or frightening.
- Technical difficulties from sensor errors, failed calibrations, and user error.

Are you and your child ready for CGM?

To help you and your family make a decision if CGM is right for your child, consider the following points:

- Are you and your child willing to check blood glucose frequently, keep records, troubleshoot, and make daily self-care decisions?
- Is your child willing to wear a device on his or her body?
- Does your child have enough body fat to wear the sensor and transmitter?
- Will your family be able to handle all the additional glucose information (glucose readings every 5 minutes) being provided?
- Is there a good support system in place to assist in handling the extra tasks added to daily diabetes care?
- Do you have time to commit to learn continuous glucose monitoring?
- Do you have a basic understanding of insulin action and carbohydrate counting?
- Will your insurance company provide CGM coverage and if not will you be able to afford this beneficial but costly device? A CGM can cost up to $1000 and sensors cost between $35-60 each.

Considering all of these things, it is important to discuss with your healthcare team if this is the right choice for your child.

Using the Information from CGM

CGM provides data in 2 ways: real time glucose with trend and retrospective data.

Trend involves the rate of change of glucose and lets you know if your glucose is rising, falling or steady. How you determine this depends on the individual device. There may be a trend graph and/or trend arrows. The 1 hour graph screen on the DexCom receiver allows you to determine what direction the glucose is trending and how quickly it may be rising or falling. The Navigator and both Medtronic devices use arrows to let you know how quickly the glucose is rising or falling.

The information involving the trend will help you to better calculate an insulin dose for carbohydrate and/or high blood glucose. If glucose is rising, you will increase the insulin dose by 10% or 20%. If it is falling, you will decrease the insulin dose by either 10% or 20%. The decision between 10% and 20% is based on how quickly the change is occurring. For example, if your daughter's blood glucose is 300 you may decide to give her a correction dose. You calculate a dose based on the sensitivity or correction factor prescribed by her healthcare team. You then look at the 1 hour trend graph on the DexCom receiver and note that her blood glucose dropped 30 mg/dL in the past 30 minutes. With this additional information, you would lower the insulin dose to prevent a low blood glucose. Conversely, if you noted her glucose rose 30 mg/dL over 30 minutes, you would add additional insulin to the dose to blunt this response.

Your healthcare team will give you more detailed algorithms that will be a starting point for making sense of glucose data and for making treatment decisions. It is important to note that you and your healthcare team may need to modify these guidelines to better fit your child.

Retrospective data lets you analyze what has happened to glucose in the past. The data stored in each CGM device can be downloaded to your computer. There are multiple options for looking at information in the form of graphs, pie charts, tables, statistical reports, and more. These options will vary by device. You will likely find that you have a favorite way of viewing the information that helps you best understand the glucose data.

Looking at this 24/7 information will allow you to look for patterns. It is best to focus on 4 or 5 days at a time and look at the most recent information, unless there are unusual circumstances, such as illness, extra exercise, travel, exams, etc., related to this time period. One of the most helpful reports to look for patterns is the 7-day overlay. A pattern is defined by similar glucose readings 2 out of 3 days. If a pattern is noted, a change in treatment strategy should be considered. Remember that it may not always be an insulin dose that needs to be changed. All reasons for high and low glucose need to be examined before making a change.

When making changes, it is important to follow these guidelines:

- Only make one change at a time
- Wait several days before making the next change
- Changes in insulin doses should be small and only made in increments of 10%

As always, discuss with your healthcare team the best way for you to interpret your child's data and make changes.

Summary

As you can see, this variety of available tools will help you to manage diabetes. With the use of blood glucose monitoring, ketone monitoring, hemoglobin A1C tests/eAG and, perhaps, continuous glucose monitoring, you and your healthcare team are provided with both the immediate and long-term information that will make caring for your child easier. You will be better able to balance insulin, food and activity so that your child lives a healthy life today and is prepared for a healthy tomorrow.

References and Resources

Nathan DM, Kuenen J, Borg R, Zheng H, Schoenfeld D, & Heine RJ, for the A1C-Derived Average Glucose (ADAG) Study Group. Translating the A1C assay into estimated average glucose values. *Diabetes Care*. 2008; 31:1473-1478.

Web sites:

- For a complete list of available diabetes monitoring products refer to the American Diabetes Association Annual Resource Guide at www.diabetes.org
- Blood glucose monitors: forecast.diabetes.org
- CGM devices: forecast.diabetes.org

7

Healthy Eating and Nutrition

At Joslin, we stress whole-family heart-healthy eating and the teaching of carbohydrate counting for diabetes self-management. Although food choices may be daunting when your family is new to diabetes, this chapter will provide you with the knowledge and skills for eating healthy foods, mindful of their impact on blood glucose levels. First, we will spend time reviewing healthy eating and dispel some of the food myths associated with diabetes. Then we will spend time reviewing carbohydrate counting, which will allow greater flexibility in managing your child's diabetes. The days when children with diabetes were restricted from eating certain foods are gone. Your child does not need to eat differently from the rest of the family and the goal is for everyone to eat healthfully.

Family Nutrition

Healthy eating is most successful when it is the routine for the entire family. All healthy eating, with or without diabetes, should focus on whole grains, lean proteins, and plenty of fruits and vegetables. Be a role model for your children — they will copy what they see parents and other family members eating. Foods that are high in sugar, empty calories, and fast foods should not replace healthy choices and should only be an occasional treat. Your job as a parent is to provide healthy food choices and listen to your child about how much he or she needs. Create a healthy food environment in your home; stack the deck in your favor by purchasing and providing healthy foods for all meals and snacks.

What is Meal Planning?

Meal planning is an important part of your child's diabetes management plan. Successful meal planning for diabetes can match your child's and family's nutrition needs, eating habits and patterns, and provide you with flexibility for the picky eater, good eater, party-goer, fast-food lover, trick-or-treater — for just about every child or teen!

A *meal plan is not a diet*. It is a guide to help you choose heart-healthy, age-appropriate meals and snacks for your child. It is important to remember that children with diabetes are children first; their nutrition needs and favorite foods will be similar to their brothers, sisters, and friends who do not have diabetes. Providing well-balanced choices does not exclude the occasional treat, and this is appropriate for all children, with or without diabetes. The meal plan should be individual to your child. Eating meals 4-5 hours apart with snacks 2-3 hours in between may work well with certain insulin regimens, while some regimens do not call for a set schedule, such as basal/bolus or pump therapy. Some families may prefer a meal plan to use as a guideline to balance their child's food with insulin and physical activity, while providing enough calories (energy) and nutrients for normal growth.

Who Helps with Your Child's Meal Planning?

A Registered Dietitian (RD) is part of your diabetes healthcare team and has special education and hospital training in the science of food and nutrition. Medical Nutrition Therapy (MNT) is the accepted term covering the information and guidance the RD provides for your family to optimize your child's diabetes management. The RD will provide nutrition education about how carbohydrates, as well as proteins, fats and fiber, impact blood glucose levels. At diagnosis you will learn nutrition survival skills. Many nutrition and food questions can arise on an ongoing basis, so making a list as they occur will ensure all your questions can be addressed at your child's scheduled follow-up appointments. Annual RD visits (more if your child is very young) help you to make the necessary adjustments at times of change such as when your child grows, as your teen stops growing, as your teen requires more calcium, or as your child or teen becomes more or less physically active. It is best to meet with a RD who has experience in the care of children with diabetes. These RD visits reinforce carbohydrate counting and healthy eating and allow a review of your child's nutrition status and blood glucose control. They will also open up all sorts of options for healthy food choices discussion.

The Meal Plan

A meal plan is individually designed to fit your child's specific needs, usual eating patterns, food preferences, activity, growth and development, and nutritional needs. Additionally, respect is paid to the individual's religious, ethnic, and cultural dietary practices. A young child generally needs 3 meals and 2-3 snacks each day. The older child should have 3 meals and 1-2 snacks daily. The number of snacks might be dependent on the insulin regime. In addition, we do not want the meals and snacks to be so far apart that your child is famished and overeats at the next meal.

There are a variety of ways to develop a meal plan. The 3 most commonly used for children with type 1 diabetes are:

1. Basic Carbohydrate Counting Meal Plan
2. Advanced Carbohydrate Counting Meal Plan
3. Exchange/Choice/Food List Meal Plan (which is used with children with type 2 diabetes or if weight loss is a goal of the child's family and healthcare team.)

Carbohydrate counting is the focus of the meal plan because it is what will affect the blood glucose the most and will determine your child's insulin needs. The better understanding you have of carbohydrate counting and portion sizes, the more flexibility you will have in your child's meal plan. All carbohydrates, and only a very minimal amount of proteins and fats, are converted to glucose. Most carbohydrates are digested within 15-60 minutes, but the presence of protein and fat can slow down the digestion.

The digestion times for nutrients are:		
Carbohydrate: 1-2 hours	Protein: 2-4 hours	Fat: 4-6 hours

Basic Carbohydrate Counting Meal Plan

This method of carbohydrate counting is used most often when a child is on 3-4 shots daily and/or eats at consistent times. The amount of carbohydrate is based on your child's daily routine and appetite. The healthcare provider will match insulin needs to the food. The family will be given a range of carbohydrate grams to be eaten at each meal or snack, such as 45-50 grams of carbohydrate at each meal and 10-15 grams at snacks.

Choosing carbohydrates from all the food groups is the basis of a healthy meal plan. The six basic food groups (meat and protein, grains, fruits, vegetables, dairy, and fats and oils) are the foundation of the meal plan. These are everyday foods you buy at the grocery store, find at home, or eat when going out. In general, a family new to diabetes will be taught both the exchange/choice meal plan followed by information on carbohydrate counting. Having a basic understanding of the carbohydrate choices/exchange list sets the foundation for choosing healthy portion sizes.

Advanced Carbohydrate Counting Meal Plan

Advanced carb counting takes your understanding of how to count carbohydrates and allows you to calculate an insulin dose based on the quantity of carbohydrates at the meal or snack and adjust the insulin based on the blood glucose. This method of insulin dosing can give increased flexibility at your child's meals and snacks. Your diabetes educator will provide you with three numbers you will need to use advanced carb counting: insulin-to-carbohydrate (I:CARB) ratio, sensitivity factor (SF), and target blood glucose or glucose range.

- **Bolus** is the insulin used to cover the carbohydrate eaten at a meal or snack or correct an elevated blood glucose.
- **Insulin-to-Carbohydrate Ratio (I:Carb)** is the amount of carbohydrate that 1 unit of rapid-acting insulin covers in your child. Your child's I:Carb will be determined by his or her total daily insulin dose (TDD). As discussed in Chapter 5: Insulin Pumps, to calculate the I:Carb, the 450 Rule can be used. Thus, if your

child's TDD is 30 units a day we divide 450 by 30 (450/30), and her I:Carb ratio is 15. So for every 15 grams of carbohydrate she eats at a meal or snack, you will give her 1 unit of rapid-acting insulin. If the total carbs at the meal is 60, you would divide by 15 and your child will need 4 units of insulin to cover the meal.

- **Sensitivity Factor (SF) (correction factor)** is how many mg/dL 1-unit of rapid-acting insulin will lower your child's blood glucose. To determine your child's SF, we again use the TDD and this time use the 1650 Rule (also discussed in Chapter 5: Insulin Pumps). We would divide 1650 by the 30 units of the TDD to calculate a SF of 55 (1650/30=55). This means that 1-unit of rapid-acting insulin would lower your child's blood glucose 55 mg/dL. This is the number we use to correct the blood glucose (BG) if it is higher or lower than desired. The correction calculation is always the same:

  (BG now) – (BG target) divided by the Sensitivity Factor =
  # of units to correct the blood glucose
- **Target Blood Glucose** is the blood glucose number or range to which we want to correct the blood glucose.

The I:CARB ratio, SF, and target BG can vary throughout the day, depending on the child's sensitivity to insulin, physical activity and daily schedule. When starting a basal/bolus insulin program, your diabetes educator will determine your child's I:CARB ratio, SF, and target blood glucose and ask you to track some data so that they can be fine-tuned to your child's plan.

How to Calculate the Insulin Needed for a Meal

Let's calculate the dose of insulin your child will need for the same meal but with different blood glucose readings. The first meal will be with a high blood glucose and the second will be with a low blood glucose.

I:CARB ratio = 1 unit of insulin for every 15 grams of carbohydrate
SF (Sensitivity Factor) = 55

Target blood glucose number is 120 mg/dL during the daytime and 150 mg/dL at bedtime

Sample Dinner Meal:	
1 cup mashed potatoes	27 grams carbs
1 tsp. margarine	0 carbs
½ cup steamed broccoli florets	0 carbs
3 oz. roasted chicken breast	0 carbs
8 oz. low-fat milk	12 grams carb
½ cup ice cream	18 grams carb
Total Number of Carbs	**57 grams carb**

First we want to determine how much rapid-acting insulin your child will need for this sample dinner meal described above.

Assume your child's pre-meal blood glucose is 220 mg/dL.

1. How many grams of carbohydrate are in this meal? *57 grams.*
2. How many units of insulin do you need to cover the carbohydrate in this meal? *3.8 units (57 gram carb/15 = 3.8 units of insulin).*
3. How many units of insulin do you need to correct for the high blood glucose? *+1.8 units (220 – 120 = 100, 100/55 = 1.8 units of insulin).*
4. What is the total number of units of insulin needed? *5.6 units (3.8 + 1.8 = 5.6 units).*

Now let's try the same meal but assume your child's blood glucose is low. The pre-meal blood glucose is 85 mg/dL

1. Insulin needed to cover the same meal above? *3.8 units.*
2. How many units of insulin do you need to correct the blood glucose? *–0.6 units (85 – 120 = –35/55 = –0.6).*
3. What is the total number of units of insulin needed? *3.2 units (3.8 + –0.6 = 3.2 units).*

Before actually starting a basal/bolus program, your educator will encourage you to practice carbohydrate counting and the calculations for a few days to reinforce the concepts.

Exchange/Choice/Food List Meal Plan

The third meal plan is the Exchange/Choice/Food List Meal Plan which focuses on the number of carbohydrates, where the carbs come from, and also provides guidance for protein and fat. Parents of young children with diabetes often worry about what their child is eating and this plan gives them direction concerning how to choose their food. This type of meal plan can also be used in combination with other carbohydrate counting methodologies when an older adolescent wants to lose weight or does not want to gain any inappropriate weight.

Most of the carbohydrate we eat comes from the following food groups: bread/starch/starchy vegetables, fruit, and dairy. Non-starchy vegetables also contain small amounts of carbohydrates, but have no significant effect on blood glucose when eaten within reasonable amounts. Foods in the meat and fat groups contain very little carbohydrate. The American

Table 7-1. Choose Your Foods: Exchange List for Diabetes

The Food Lists	CHO (grams)	Protein (grams)	Fat (grams)	Calories
Carbohydrate				
Starch: breads, cereals and grains, starchy vegetables, crackers, snacks, and beans, peas, and lentils	15	0 – 3	0 – 1	80
Fruits	15	–	–	60
Milk				
Fat-Free, low-fat, 1%	12	8	0 – 3	100
Reduced-fat, 2%	12	8	5	120
Whole	12	8	8	160
Sweets, Desserts, and Other Carbohydrates	15	varies	varies	varies
Non-Starchy Vegetables	5	2	–	25
Meat & Meat Substitutes				
Lean	–	7	0 – 3	45
Medium-Fat	–	7	4 – 7	75
High-Fat	–	7	8+	100
Plant-based proteins	varies	7	varies	varies
Fat	–	–	5	45
Alcohol	varies	–	–	100

Dietetic Association publishes what is called an exchange list, which identifies the amount of carbohydrate, protein, fat, and calories in many foods. In the most recent update of the exchange list, the title has been changed to *Choose Your Foods: Exchange List for Diabetes* (see Table 7-1), and has an additional carbohydrate list that includes sweets, dessert, and other carbohydrates. The list in Table 7-1 represents the amount of carbohydrate, protein, and fat in a predetermined serving size for each food group.

For example, 1 carbohydrate serving of starch, fruit, or starchy vegetables and legumes all contains approximately 15 grams of carbohydrate. 1 to 2 servings of non-starchy vegetables do not have to be counted, as they have a very small affect on blood glucose due to their low carb content and that some of the carb comes from fiber.

Food Lists

Each carbohydrate food list records how much of each food is needed to equal 15 grams of carbohydrate. For example, 3 cups of air-popped popcorn or one-half of a grapefruit each contain 15 grams of carbohydrate. Therefore, foods found on each of the food lists can be substituted or exchanged with other food from the same list. The exchange/choice/list system allows for a meal plan to be consistent while offering a variety of food choices. Examples of the food lists with amounts equal to 1 choice are listed in Table 7-2. This is a very basic list and is usually supplemented with carbohydrate-counting books, which list the grams of carbohydrate in a single serving of a wide variety of foods, and are available at bookstores to make carbohydrate counting easier. If you are using this type of meal planning, your dietitian will develop a meal plan that tells you how much of each of the food groups your child should eat at each meal and snack. Your dietitian will make this plan based on your child's normal eating schedule, age and weight, nutritional needs, activity level, and the amount of insulin he or she takes.

Keep in mind the exchange/choice/food list is an average portion size and due to the large variety of choices that we have on the market today, not all foods are equal. For instance, if you are making your child's lunch

Table 7-2. Examples of Food Lists

Carbohydrate = 15 grams carb per serving

Breads, Cereals & Grains	Beans	Starchy Vegetables	Fruit
1 slice bread	½ cup beans or peas (garbanzo, pinto, kidney, white, lentils, black, black-eyed peas, etc.)	½ C corn	6 ½ oz orange
¼ large bagel (1 oz)	⅓ cup baked beans	½ C green peas	¼ C dried fruit
6″ tortilla		1 C winter squash	1 ¼ C watermelon
½ 6″ pita bread		3 oz potato (baked, boiled, roasted)	1 ¼ C strawberries
½ English muffin		2 oz. Sweet potato	1 C raspberries
½ C cooked cereal		½ C mashed potato	¾ C black or blueberries
¾ C unsweetened dry cereal		½ C mashed sweet potato	½ grapefruit
⅓ C cooked rice or pasta			½ C (5 ½ oz.) mango
2 slices reduced-calorie bread			½ C fruit juice
1 C soup			17 grapes
Crackers/snacks	**Milk**	**Desserts/Sweets**	3 ½ oz banana
3 C air-popped popcorn	1 C milk (FF, skim, 1%, 2% whole, Lactaid)	1 oz angel cake	1 C melon
18–20 mini pretzels	6 oz Light yogurt	2″ sq unfrosted cake	15 cherries
5–8 pretzels twist	8 oz plain yogurt	2″ sq brownie	1 C pineapple
6 whole grain crackers	½ C evaporated milk	2 small cookies	4 oz pc fresh fruit
3 graham crackers	⅓ C dry fat-free milk	½ C ice cream	
2 rice cakes, 4″ across		¼ C sherbet/sorbet	
17 potato chips		1 Tbsp jam or jelly	
10 tortilla chips		1 Tbsp honey	

and the meal plan is 2 starches, 2 proteins, 1 fruit, and 1 milk, the meal could look like this:

- Sliced chicken sandwich
  - White bread 2 slices = 22 grams carb, 0 fiber
  - Whole grain bread 2 slices = 36 grams carb, 2 gram fiber (36 – 2 gram fiber = 34 grams carb)
- 2 oz sliced chicken
- ½ cup fruit salad (15 grams carb)
- 8 oz of low fat milk (12 grams carb)

The type of bread could make a big difference in the total carbs at the meal. The lunch made with the white bread would have 49 grams of carb and the lunch made with whole grain bread would have 61 grams of carb. Eating the whole grain is the healthiest choice but might require more insulin.

Free Foods

Free foods are those with less than 25 calories and 5 grams of carbohydrate per serving. These foods should not cause blood glucose spikes and are considered good fillers as needed to compliment the meal plan. Non-starchy vegetables are full of fiber and vitamins. These foods have very little carbohydrate and minimal effect on blood glucose levels. A few examples:

- Non-starchy Vegetables: asparagus, artichoke, bell peppers (red, orange, green, and yellow), broccoli, cauliflower, carrots, celery, cucumbers, lettuce, green beans, mushrooms, spinach, tomatoes, etc.
- Olives
- Pickles
- Sugar-free gelatin or popsicles
- No- or low-calorie drinks

Healthy Snacking Ideas

Snacks are an important part of your child's meal plan. They help keep your child's blood glucose in balance and are often necessary for children to eat enough calories throughout the day to grow. Children often think of snack foods as junk foods such as chips, crackers, fruit snacks and cookies; however, fresh fruits, vegetables and healthy fat foods should also be included as snacks. These snacks will help your child develop healthy eating habits for life.

15-Gram Carbohydrate Snack Ideas	
Fruit	**Dried Fruit**
Apple, small (4 oz)	Banana Flakes, 3 Tbsp
Applesauce, unsweetened (4 oz)	Dates, 4 medium (total 1 oz)
Apricots, fresh, 2 medium (2 oz each)	Fig, 1 medium
Avocado, 1 medium (7 oz)	Prunes (dried plums), 3 medium
Banana, small (4 oz)	Raisins, 1½ Tbsp (¾ oz)
Berries (blue/boysenberry), ¾ cup	Yogurt Raisins, 1 ounce
Cantaloupe, 1 cup (5 oz)	**Crackers/Cookies/Snack Food**
Carambola (star fruit), 4 medium	Animal Crackers, 8 – 10*
Cherries, 12	Bread, whole wheat, 1 slice
Clementine, 3 small	English muffin, whole wheat, ½
Fruit cups/salads, ½ cup	Whole wheat Fig Newton, 1
Grapefruit, ½, 10 oz (6 oz flesh)	Ginger snaps, 3
Grapes, 10-15 (4 oz)	Graham, 2½″ sq., 3
Guava, 4 oz	Goldfish crackers, 43*
Honey dew, 1 cup (6 oz)	Mini-flavored rice cakes, 6 (check flavor)
Kiwi, 1 large (4 oz)	Oyster crackers, 60 small or 30 large
Kumquats, 5 medium (3½ oz)	Popcorn, 3 cups air-popped or low fat
Lychees, 8 fruit (5 oz)	Pretzels, 2 rods, 30 sticks or ¾oz
Nectarine, 1 medium (5 oz)	Rice cakes, 2
Mandarin, 1 large (6 oz)	Rice Krispy Treat, 1
Mango, 4 oz flesh	Ritz Bits mini sandwiches, 12**
Orange, 1 small (5 oz w/skin)	Sandwich cracker w/cheese or peanut butter, 4*
Papaya, 1 cup cubed (5 oz)	Saltine-type crackers, 4
Passion fruit, 3 medium (4 oz)	Teddy Grahams, 15
Peach, 1 large (6 oz)	Tortilla chips, 6 – 12 (1 ounce)**
Pear, 1 small (4 oz)	Vanilla Wafers, 5
Persimmons, 3 oz	**Breakfast Foods**
Pineapple, ¾ cup (4 oz)	Bagel, ½ of a two oz bagel
Plantain, 2 oz	French toast, low fat, 1 slice
Plum, 1 large (4 oz)	Granola, ¼ cup*
Pomegranates, 1 fruit (5 oz)	Hot cereal, ½ cup or 1 package
Quince, 1 medium (3½ oz)	Milk, low fat, 8 oz
Raspberries, 1 cup (4 oz)	Muffin small, 1 oz, 1*
Strawberries, 1½ cup (8 oz)	Pancake, 4-inch, 2
Tangerine, 1 medium (4 oz)	Whole grain cereal, ¾ – 1 cup
Ugli fruit, 2 fruits (5 oz each)	Whole grain waffle, 1
Watermelon, 1 small slice (8 oz)	Yogurt, plain, low fat, 8 oz
Items marked with an asterisk have about 5 grams (*) or 10 grams (**) of fat per serving and should be use sparingly.	

Healthy Homemade Snacks Examples

- 1-2 slices of whole wheat bread (you can toast the bread)
  - Plus slices of lean luncheon meat (add lettuce, tomato) OR
  - Plus slices of low fat cheese OR
  - Plus peanut butter (and fruit spread or blueberries or apple or banana) OR
  - Plus tuna
- 1 to 1½ cups whole grain cereal, 4-6 oz skim or low fat milk
- ½ cup plain yogurt, ½ cup frozen blueberries or fruit of choice, sweetened with sugar substitute
- Whole wheat English Muffin, tablespoon of pizza or tomato sauce, ½ oz shredded cheese
- Graham crackers with natural peanut butter
- Ants on a log – celery sticks with peanut butter and raisins on top
- Apples or pears with peanut butter or 1 oz cheese
- Whole wheat crackers with low fat cream cheese or natural peanut butter or egg
- ½ – 1 cup cut up fruit
- Raw vegetable sticks with low-fat yogurt dip, cottage cheese or hummus
- Bruschetta: Melba toast, chopped tomatoes, little olive oil
- Smoothie: low fat yogurt blended with fresh or frozen fruit
- Cottage cheese with fresh, frozen, or canned fruit
- Baked or tortilla chips and bean dip or salsa
- Banana rolled in peanut butter, wrap in wax paper, freeze overnight
- Apple or pear, core, add a little bit of water, cinnamon, and Splenda, microwave for 2 minutes

Individualization Allows for Flexibility

To be effective, a nutrition plan must be flexible so that it is realistic for your child and your family. Children's lives, although routine at times, often incorporate changes in plans, special events, and periods when eating habits change. By individualizing a plan for your child, all of these non-routine events or periods can be managed successfully.

Special Occasions and Parties

Birthday parties are fun and very much part of growing up for most of us. You will be happy to learn that foods at birthday parties do not cause most children's blood glucose to be exceptionally high. Why? Most children are more interested in running and playing with their friends than the cake and ice cream. On the other hand, children may be so happy to eat foods like cake and ice cream, usually limited at home, that they may clean their plate. Learn how your child reacts by experience, and make adjustments. Yes, a chocolate cupcake at a party is OK! It would provide on average 20-25 grams of carb. Once children reach the age of 4 or 5, a friend's birthday party is very important and your child can and should participate and have fun.

The Trick-or-Treater

Halloween means candy and probably stress for you, as parents of a child with diabetes. But stress reduction is possible. Consider making some changes for all children in the family:

- Let your children go trick-or-treating; then let them trade their candy for money, a new outfit, a special outing with the family, or a special toy from their favorite store.
- Make a big deal about dressing up in a favorite costume, letting your child decide what he or she wants to be.
- Have a neighborhood Halloween party where you decide what is being served.
- Provide a healthy alternative at your house or even a small toy or trinket such as crayons, coloring books, Halloween pencils, etc.
- Ask neighbors and friends to give your children sugar-free gum, sugar-free soda, granola bars, small bags of pretzels, popcorn, or baked chips.
- Go to special programs for children with diabetes in your community — often sponsored by organizations such as your local American Diabetes Association affiliate.

- Have your children pick their favorite items from the candy they have collected and then include 1 piece daily at lunch or dinner for the next few weeks. Give away the rest. That way, no one in the family will be eating candy simply because it's there.

Dining Out

Eating out as a family or going to a fast food restaurant with a friend is a special occasion for most children. Many fast food and other restaurants have nutrition information available either posted in the restaurants, on the menu, or available via the internet. By mastering portions and carb counting at home, you will be able to estimate the amount of carbs while dining out. Remember, if you are not sure how many carbs are in the meal, underestimate and then check your child's blood glucose in 2-3 hours. You can always add more insulin if necessary.

The Picky Eater

A picky eater will eat just a few foods and does not want to try new foods. Almost every child goes through a stage like this. Some continue this pattern throughout life. Some like the extra attention they get by being picky, while others really do hate the taste of certain foods. What can you do? Try not to worry if your child wants to eat the same food every meal for weeks (only bananas and peanut butter sandwiches), as most children grow out of this stage. Do your job by providing healthy foods at regular times. Keep in mind that children often need 10 or more exposures to a new food before they accept it, so be persistent!

- Introduce a new food in a neutral manner. For younger children, talk about the food's color, shape, size, aroma and texture, but not about whether it tastes good. A few examples could be:
  - Decorate the plate with fruit or vegetables slices.
  - Top off a bowl of cereal with berries or make a smiley face on waffles or hot cereal.
- Your child may want to touch and smell new food before tasting it. For pre-teens and teens, talk about the nutrition benefit, the recipe, and the origin of the food.

- Make sure you are eating the foods you want your child to eat. Set a good example and eat fruits and/or vegetables at your meals and snacks. Children often mimic their parents, so the more frequently you eat a food, the more likely your child may eventually try it.
- Get your child involved with food shopping and preparation. The child may get more excited about a new food if he or she helps to pick it out and serve it to the family.
- Don't overload your child with too many new foods at once. Place a small portion of the new food on your child's plate next to foods she or he already enjoys.
- Some children are just too busy to think about food. Try to slow things down prior to meals. Phone calls, texting, and homework can all wait until after the meal.
- Make the new food fun and interesting. Try serving it with a dipping sauce or cutting it into different shapes. Younger children may like to name the dish (moon juice for milk, trees for broccoli, clouds for mashed potatoes, etc.). Find an interesting fact about the food and share it at mealtime.
- Have only 1 food your child likes as a back-up for when he or she refuses to eat. Suggestions: cereal with milk, peanut butter or grilled cheese sandwich, or yogurt with fruit. Make it simple. If you are concerned about your child's growth, ask your diabetes healthcare team if your child is growing well. This is the true test if he or she is getting enough to eat.
- If your child tries the food but states he or she does not like it, thank him or her for trying the food. For instance, if you served a new vegetable and your child tried it and said "I don't like it," your response could be "Thank you for trying it. I am so proud of you. Maybe you will like it when you get bigger."
- Try not to make eating a battleground and ask your RD for more ideas!

The Good Eater?

Some children overeat and diabetes can often make this worse because of the focus on what and how much your child with diabetes is eating. If your child seems to be overeating, it may be for a good reason, as hunger can:

- mean your child is in a growth spurt and needs more calories,
- be a symptom of low blood glucose; make sure to check your child's blood glucose,
- reflect high blood glucose and a need for more insulin; make sure to check your child's blood glucose.

Consider the difference between true hunger and boredom. Have low-calorie foods available if boredom seems to be the stimulus rather than true hunger. It is difficult to eat while engaged in activities, such as playing outside, running, building models, and playing sports. If the constant hunger persists, speak to your healthcare team to review your child's dietary intake and insulin.

Tools for Healthy Eating

Dietary Guidelines for Americans

The United States Department of Agriculture (USDA) created Dietary Guidelines for Americans in 2005, giving science-based advice on food and physical activity choices for health. The Dietary Guidelines describe a healthy diet as one that:

- Emphasizes fruits, vegetables, whole grains, and fat-free or low-fat milk and milk products;
- Includes lean meats, poultry, fish, beans, eggs, and nuts; and
- Is low in saturated fats, trans fats, cholesterol, salt (sodium), and added sugars.

The revised USDA food pyramid (MyPyramid) is used as a guide to healthy eating and is based on the 2005 Dietary Guidelines for Americans. There are different versions of MyPyramid that are based on age groups and the web site even allows you to customize your pyramid based on individual activity level, height, and weight. The revised

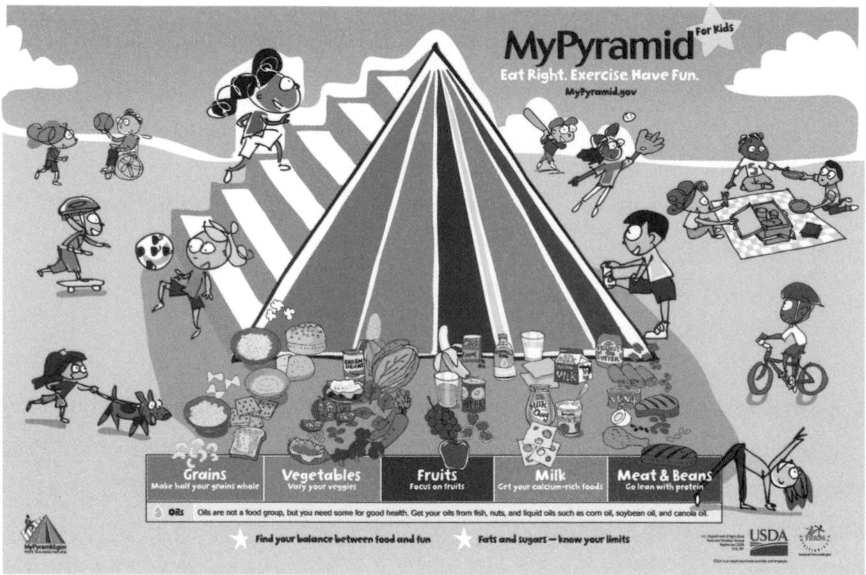

FIGURE 7-1. USDA MyPyramid for Kids (3)

pyramids also emphasize the importance of exercise. These recommendations are for the general public over the age of 2 and suggest that some foods from each of the following food groups be eaten daily to achieve a well balanced meal plan. From the size of the food group's color stripe, you can see which foods are encouraged to be eaten in greater quantities:

- Grains
- Vegetables
- Fruits
- Milk
- Meats & Beans

While MyPyramid is a great visual tool, it is important to look further than the pictures for suggestions on the food groups. There are many ways to eat healthy — one may be best for your family and another for your neighbor. See the web sites listed at the end of the chapter to look up additional information about the pyramids along with tools and some fun activities. Remember, when looking at suggestions for food groups, serving sizes are different at various ages. Two servings of fruit for a 2 year old

Table 7-3. Suggested Portion Sizes for Children

Food Type	Ages 1-2 years	Ages 3-5 years	Ages 6-12 years
Milk	½ cup	¾ cup	1 cup
Fruit or Vegetable Juice	¼ cup	½ cup	½ cup
Fruit or Vegetable	¼ cup total	½ cup total	¾ cup total
Bread	½ slice	½ slice	1 slice
Dry Cereal (volume or weight)	¼ cup or ⅓ oz	⅓ cup or ½ oz	¾ cup or 1 oz
Pasta, Cooked Cereal, Noodles	¼ cup	¼ cup	½ cup
Lean Meat, Fish, Poultry, Cheese	1 oz.	1.5 oz	2 oz
Eggs	½ egg	¾ egg	1 egg
Peanut Butter or other Nut Butters	2 Tbsp	3 Tbsp	4 Tbsp
Yogurt	½ cup	¾ cup	1 cup
Cooked Beans or Legumes	¼ cup	⅓ cup	½ cup

will be smaller than 2 servings of fruit for a 10 year old. Table 7-3 lists portion sizes for some common foods.

The Plate Method

A very handy tool used in nutrition education is the plate method to reinforce healthy portions and a balanced meal. Picture a small dinner plate and divide that plate in half. Half the plate should be filled with non-starchy vegetables such as salad, carrots, broccoli, or green beans. Then cut the other side of the plate in half and one quarter is for the carbohydrate food such as mashed potato, rice or pasta and the other quarter is for the protein such as baked chicken, fish, or lean meats. On the side of the plate also include a small piece of fruit and an 8 oz glass of low-fat milk.

What can healthy foods do for you?

Everyone needs to eat healthy foods, rich in vitamins and minerals:

- for energy to learn, play and live
- to manage blood glucose

- for proper bodily function
- to maintain a healthful weight
- for children and teens to grow at a healthy rate and develop strong bones and muscles
- for normal ongoing body maintenance, even for adults who are no longer growing
- to help prevent diet related diseases

Macronutrients

The energy in our food comes from sources known as macronutrients. The three macronutrients are carbohydrates, protein, and fat. The caloric content of the macronutrients are listed in Table 7-4.

Nutrition guidelines recommend having a balanced intake of these 3 macronutrients. Recommendations for your child's caloric needs are individualized based on age, activity, weight, height, and management goals. The national recommendations in Table 7-5 are based on the Dietary Reference Intakes (DRI)* and will be referred to often in this chapter.

Table 7-4. Caloric Content of Macronutrients

Macronutrient	Calories per gram
Carbohydrates	4
Protein	4
Fat	9

Table 7-5. Recommended Ranges for Macronutrients

Macronutrient	Percent of Total Calories
Carbohydrate	45–65%
Protein	15–20%
Fat	20–30%

Carbohydrates (CHO)

The main job of a carbohydrate is to provide energy to your cells in the form of glucose or sugar. Carbohydrates are the starch and sugars found in foods, with the simplest forms of carbohydrate being glucose, fructose, and lactose. All starches and sugars break down into glucose in our body and become the primary fuel for our brain and central nervous system. Over

* The Dietary Reference Intake (DRI) is a set of nutrition recommendations for the general public (US and Canada) from the Institute of Medicine (IOM) of the US National Academy of Sciences. It was created in 1997 to broaden existing guidelines used by health professionals. (6)

the age of 1 year, it is recommended that no one have less than 130 grams/day. Carbohydrates consist of:

- Starches, found in pasta, breads, cereals, potatoes, peas, lentils, and beans
- Natural sugars, found in milk, vegetables, and fruits
- Added sugars, found in syrups, jams and sweets, along with many other packaged foods

There are a number of sugars that are added to sweeten our foods. Some examples that you might find on food labels are: sucrose, glucose, fructose, dextrose, lactose, maltose, honey, corn syrup, molasses, fruit juice concentrates, and high fructose corn syrup. Most of these simple sugars are not providing any nutritional benefit and should be limited.

Whole grains are beneficial to the heart and choosing them for the family will benefit everyone's health. A whole grain includes all three layers of the grain: the bran, endosperm, and germ. Together, these provide fiber, vitamins, and phytonutrients (health-protective substances in plant foods) which help protect against heart disease. Fiber can also help avoid spikes in blood glucose. "Refined grain" is often used to refer to products that use only part of the grain (endosperm) and are missing many of the nutrients that the whole grain contains. These may be labeled as "enriched" flour or grains on the ingredients list. Examples include white bread, sugary cereals, cookies, or regular crackers. It is always preferred to buy the version with whole grains — look for "whole" listed first in the ingredients or a picture of whole grain stamped on the side of the box.

Proteins

The body uses protein for growth and energy; protein is considered the building block for muscles and bones. Protein comes from both animal and plant sources: meat, fish, dairy products, beans, peas, lentils, and eggs. Vegetables and starches have small amounts of protein, while animal sources have greater amounts of protein. Recommended protein intake is based on body weight and is set at DRI of 0.8 g/kg. Based on this recommendation, a young person weighing 100 pounds (45 kg) will need 36 grams of protein a day to meet his or her needs, which is very easy to achieve. For instance, an 8 oz glass of milk, 3 oz chicken breast, ½ cup green beans, and ½ cup mashed potatoes provides approximately 35 grams of protein.

When your body breaks down protein, it turns into smaller parts called amino acids, which are used for many functions in the body. The waste products made from the protein breakdown are filtered by the kidneys. High protein meal plans can put additional stress on your child's kidneys because they work to get rid of these waste-products. Joslin encourages our patients not to eat more than 2 grams of protein per kilogram (body weight) per day. As in the example above, a 100 pound (45 kg) person would have a suggested upper limit of 90 grams of protein per day.

In addition, high protein meal plans are typically high in total fat, with most of the fat being saturated and not heart healthy fat. If a child is eating a high protein/high fat meal plan, he or she may be excluding nutrient-dense foods such as fresh fruits and whole grains.

Does more protein mean bigger muscles?

Many of our teen and young adult athletes ask whether, if they eat more protein, they can build bigger muscles. Excess protein intake does not mean more muscles. Muscles are developed by physical activity, in addition to healthy eating and management of diabetes. For our athletes that wish to increase strength and muscle mass, we recommend visiting with an Exercise Physiologist to determine an individual exercise plan to meet their needs. Generally, it is beneficial to replace protein stores after strength workouts, which is incorporated into their daily requirements. This post-workout snack might be a turkey sandwich and a glass of milk, a nut-filled protein bar, or even a typical dinner that includes one of the following heart-healthy protein sources:

- Lean cuts of meats (beef, pork, veal, chicken, and turkey)
- Fish, eggs, and low fat cheese
- Dried peas, beans, and legumes (kidney, white, split, etc.)
- Soy products like tofu, tempeh (tofu and brown rice), and veggie burgers
- Nuts and nut butters, especially almonds, walnuts and cashews

Fats

Fats are essential in maintaining healthy hair, skin, and body temperature, and promoting healthy cell function. Fats also help to store excess energy in the body. There are many sources of fat in the diet. Researchers have found some fats are healthy for hearts (monounsaturated), while others such as saturated and trans-fats can lead to high cholesterol levels and increased risk of heart disease. Cholesterol is a waxy, fat-like substance made in the liver. It is present in some of the food you eat, but blood cholesterol levels are most affected by the types of fats you eat.

Types of Dietary Fat

The following lists the multiple types of fats in our diets. Polyunsaturated fats, omega-3 fatty acids, and monounsaturated fats are healthier for your heart than saturated and trans fats.

- *Polyunsaturated fats* are a good choice and have many health benefits. Sources are usually liquid at room temperature and include: sunflower oil, corn oil, and sesame oil.
- *Omega-3 fatty acids* are polyunsaturated fats found in fish, flax, and walnuts. Omega-3 fats protect the heart, so recommendations are to eat foods high in Omega-3 fatty acids, 2-3 times a week.
- *Monounsaturated fats* are one of the healthiest fats and help to lower cholesterol and blood pressure. Sources include: canola oil, olive oil, peanut oil, avocado, and nuts.
- *Saturated fats* increase cholesterol and are not healthy for the heart. Sources include: red meats, butter, cheese, whole milk, palm or coconut oil, and shortenings. Less than 10% of total energy intake should be from saturated fat.
- *Trans fats* are found in products that are hydrogenated. Sources include mostly processed and fast foods: bakery products, stick margarine, and fried foods. Pay attention to the ingredients in packaged foods and look for the word "hydrogenated." All food companies are now required to list the amount of *trans* fat on the nutrition label. Try to avoid trans fat as much as possible as it has negative effects on cholesterol and blood pressure.

Vitamins and Minerals

Vitamins and minerals are important for growth, good vision, healthy skin and hair, strong bones, and formation of blood cells. It is important to make sure your child's meal plan is well balanced and is adequate in vitamins and minerals to ensure normal growth and development.

- **Calcium** is a mineral that helps develop strong bones and teeth. It also helps your child's heart and nerves to function, which is why it is important to include calcium-rich foods as part of the meal plan. Great sources of calcium include: milk (low-fat is best), fortified soy or rice milk, yogurt, cheese, leafy green vegetables, and tofu. If your child does not eat or drink dairy products, he or she may need supplementation of calcium and vitamin D.

Table 7-6. Dietary Reference Intakes (DRI) for Calcium

Age	Calcium Intake (mg/day)	Age	Calcium Intake (mg/day)
0–6 months	210	9–18 yrs	1300
7–12 months	270	19–50 yrs	1000
1–3 yrs	500	50+ yrs	1200
4–8 yrs	800		

- **Vitamin D** is also very important in bone health; it helps the body absorb calcium and phosphorus. Fortified milk and cereals are good sources of vitamin D. The body can synthesize vitamin D when exposed to sunlight 20-30 minutes a day, but recent studies have suggested that due to varied seasons and use of sunscreen, many Americans are deficient. The Adequate Intake (AI) for Vitamin D (from birth to 50 years) is currently 5 mg per day or 200 IU. Due to reported deficiencies, the American Academy of Pediatrics (AAP) has increased its recommendation to 400 IU per day for all infants, children, and adolescents. There is much debate in the medical community; check with your dietitian for the most recent recommendations.

- **Vitamins C and E** have antioxidant properties that may help prevent heart disease. Requirements are generally met through dietary intake.
- **Zinc** is a mineral that can be lost in the urine when high blood glucose promotes increased urine output. It is important for growth and some children with diabetes may require a supplement to meet their needs. Food sources include whole grains, red meat, seafood, and some fortified grains.
- **Sodium** is also a mineral and has been linked to high blood pressure. Sodium intake should be limited to 2,300 mg/day. The average American consumes 2-3 times the amount of salt recommended. Salt in foods we eat (chips, crackers, sauces, fast foods) contributes a significant amount of sodium — even if you never use a saltshaker. Always encourage your family and child to taste their food before they use the saltshaker. A good strategy is to leave the saltshaker in the kitchen; if your child wants salt he or she has to go get the saltshaker, add it to the food and then return it to the kitchen.

There is no current evidence that people with diabetes would benefit from additional vitamin or mineral supplementation, compared to the general population. A multivitamin supplement may be suggested if your child's dietary intake lacks variety or if your child is not incorporating certain food groups. When choosing vitamins, avoid mega doses and look for an age appropriate multi-vitamin with minerals.

Water

Water is the most important nutrient of all! It makes up two-thirds of our body weight, cools our body as needed and helps remove toxins and waste. It is important to drink enough water every day and to get extra water when it is hot outside or when physically active. It is recommended to drink at least six 8 oz glasses of water daily; milk and sugar-free drinks count towards your child's fluid intake but plain water tops them all.

Dietary Fiber

Dietary fiber comes from the part of plant foods that is not absorbed into the body. Fiber in the meal plan supplies bulk and roughage, which helps to keep you feeling full, and helps to keep the digestive system moving. Increased fiber intake slows digestion of food, and therefore can help prevent spikes in blood glucose. Be sure to drink plenty of water when increasing fiber intake.

Dietary fiber is divided into 2 types:

1. **Soluble fiber** is found in oats, beans (peas, soybeans, pinto, etc.), rye, chia, barley, fruits (apples, berries, etc.), vegetables (broccoli, carrots, etc.), and seeds. It helps lower cholesterol levels.
2. **Insoluble fiber** is found in wheat bran, most whole grains, nuts, and vegetables. It helps prevent constipation.

Table 7-7. Dietary Fiber Recommended Intake

Age (years)	DRI for Males (grams/day)	DRI for Females (grams/day)
1–3	19	19
4–9	25	25
9–13	31	26
14–50	38	26
>50	30	21

Alcohol

As parents, you know the legal drinking age in the United States is 21 years. However, in reality, many adolescents and young adults are faced with alcohol in many situations. It is important for you to talk to your child to make sure he or she knows the facts about alcohol in general and combined with diabetes in particular. Alcohol lowers the blood glucose and this can be very dangerous. The liver processes alcohol; it is also the organ that releases stored glucose in the event of a low blood glucose. The liver can do one thing at a time; if it is too busy metabolizing the alcohol, then it will not release the glucose to help prevent the low blood glucose. Drinking alcoholic beverages that contain too much sugar (such as liqueurs or drink mixes) is not recommended because they will cause a high blood glucose.

Remember, when drinking alcohol:

- Check blood glucose often
- Include a snack prior to sleeping
- Never drive or get in a car with someone drinking
- Drink in moderation (1-2 drinks per day)
  - One alcohol-containing drink is defined as:
    - 12 oz beer
    - 5 oz wine or
    - 1½ oz distilled spirits

Sweeteners and Sugar Substitutes

There are many food products available today that use sweeteners and sugar substitutes that do not raise the blood glucose. These are called non-nutritive sweeteners, or artificial sweeteners, and contain an insignificant amount of calories or carbohydrate. There are six sugar substitutes approved by the Food and Drug Administration for use in foods and drinks:

- Saccharin (Sucaryl, Sugar Twin, Sweet'N Low, Sweet Twin)
- Aspartame (Equal, NatraTaste, NutraSweet)
- Acesulfame potassium or Acesulfame-K (Sunette, Sweet One)
- Neotame
- Sucralose (Splenda)
- Rebiana (Truvia)

We are often asked how much of these sweeteners are safe to consume. All six of the sugar substitutes listed have an established safety level, called the Acceptable Daily Intake (ADI). ADI is the amount of a food additive that can be safely eaten every day over your child's lifetime without causing harm. No studies have shown that sugar substitutes cause brain tumors, cancer, or other health problems. For adults and children alike, it is safe to consume non-nutritive sweeteners in the context of a healthy, well-balanced meal plan. If you think a sweetener has any side effects on your child, talk with your healthcare provider.

Do keep in mind that it is recommended to limit the intake of diet sodas containing phosphoric acid to prevent tooth decay and weakening of bones. This happens when the phosphoric acid in most sodas erodes tooth enamel and binds with calcium in the intestinal track to prevent absorption.

Sugar Alcohols

Sugar alcohols are another form of sweetener but they are not the same as sugar substitutes. Typical sugar alcohols are sorbitol, mannitol, maltitol, hydrogenated starch hydrolysate (HSH), and xylitol. These sweeteners are partially absorbed in the intestine; this means they do have some calories and carbohydrates, and may have some effect on blood glucose. Sugar alcohols are commonly found in products such as candies, which may be reported to be sugar-free, and many of the low-carb foods on the market today. Be aware — these sweeteners can cause gas, diarrhea, and stomach upset.

Tools for Nutritional Management of Diabetes

Meal planning and carbohydrate (carb) counting is most successful when it becomes the routine for the entire family. In this next section we will review some of the different tools used in meal planning.

Carb counting can be challenging in our society due to the sheer variety of available foods on the market today. Food labels are the best source of information and provide the most accurate information for a specific food. It was determined in the Diabetes Control and Complications Trial (DCCT) that six nutritional factors contribute to better blood glucose control. They are as follows:

- Following a meal plan
- Avoiding snacking in-between meals and snacks

- Avoiding over treating hypoglycemia (low blood glucose)
- Quick treatment of high blood glucoses
- Adjusting insulin at meals to match the carbohydrate
- Consistency of overnight snacks

The DCCT results confirmed what Elliott P. Joslin said in 1935, "In teaching patients their diet, I lay emphasis first on carbohydrate values, and teach to a few only the value of protein and fat." If most people concentrate on the carb content in their food and match their insulin dose accordingly, they should be able to achieve the glycemic control they desire. However, for overall health, it is important that the protein and fat content of your child's meal plan is heart healthy and nutritionally balanced.

Reading a Food Label

For diabetes management in children, there are four key areas to review on food labels. Here is what you should look for:

1. Serving Size
    a. Listed in both household measurement and by weight
2. Total Carbohydrate
    a. Compared to all other nutrients, carbohydrates raise blood glucose the most. How many grams of carbohydrate do you aim for at each meal?
    b. 1 carb choice/exchange = 15 grams carbohydrate
    c. Dietary Fiber can be subtracted from Total Carbohydrate. Choose foods with at least 3 grams of fiber per serving. Foods with 1-2 grams of fiber per 100 calories are considered good sources of fiber.
    d. Sugar Alcohols are commonly used in sugar-free products. Subtract half of the sugar alcohols from Total Carbohydrate. For example if there were 10 grams of sugar alcohol in a product, you would subtract 5 grams from the Total Carbohydrate.
3. Total Fat
    a. Fat should be limited to help control weight and reduce your risk for heart disease. Low fat foods have no more than 3 grams of fat per serving.

   b. Saturated Fat: Look for less than 1 gram per serving
   c. Trans Fat: Look for 0 grams per serving
4. Sodium
   a. Low sodium foods have no more than 140 milligrams of sodium per serving. Choose these often.

The food label will provide nutrition information, but keep in mind the food label is required by law to list the minimum "servings per package" that are in the package. To avoid violating consumer protection laws against selling underweight packages, many manufacturers deliberately overfill their individually packaged foods. As a result, individual portion packages often contain more food than the nutrition label indicates. Thus your portion could be higher in carbs than anticipated.

Foods that do not come with food labels are often the healthiest foods and the ones that are more challenging to count. Many families have shared with us that they eat less healthy foods after their child is diagnosed with diabetes because they do not know how to count the carbohydrates in fresh fruit or homemade healthy snacks. They find themselves buying all the individual snack options available on the market, and as a consequence, their child no longer eats some of his or her favorite healthy foods. This is where a food scale can be handy, because once you have weighed your child's favorite fruits a few times, you will be able to estimate its carbs. Then, when you are out of the house, you'll feel confident to provide insulin to cover the food.

Whole Grain Cereal

Nutrition Facts

Serving Size 1 cup (53g/1.9 oz.)

Amount Per Serving	
Calories 190	**Calories from Fat 25**
	% Daily Value**
Total Fat 3g*	5%
Saturated Fat 0g	0%
Trans Fat 0g	
Cholesterol 0mg	0%
Sodium 95mg	4%
Potassium 300mg	9%
Total Carbohydrate 36g	12%
Dietary Fiber 8g	32%
Soluble Fiber 3g	
Insoluble Fiber 5g	
Sugars 13g	
Protein 9g	32%

Vitamin A 0% • Vitamin C 0%
Calcium 4% • Iron 10%
Phosphorus 10% • Magnesium 10%
Copper 8%

*Amount in Cereal. One half cup of fat free milk contributes an additional 40 calories, 65mg sodium, 6g total carbohydrates (6g sugars), and 4g protein
** Percent Daily Values are based on a 2,000 calories diet. Your daily values may be higher or lower depending on your calorie needs

	Calories	2,000	2,500
Total Fat	Less Than	65g	80g
Sat. Fat	Less Than	20g	25g
Cholesterol	Less Than	300mg	300mg
Sodium	Less Than	2,400mg	2,400mg
Potassium		3,500mg	3,500mg
Total Carbohydrate		300g	375g
Dietary Fiber		25g	30g
Protein		50g	65g

Calories per gram:
Fat 9 • Carbohydrate 4 • Protein 4

INGREDIENTS: Soy Grits, Hard Red Winter Wheat, Long Grain Brown Rice, Whole Grain Oats, Barley, Rye, Buckwhaet, Sesame Seeds, Evaporated Cane Juice Syrup, Corn Meal, Corn Flour, Soy Protein, Wheat Bran, Oat Flour, Corn Bran, Honey, Natural Flavors, Calcium Carbonate, Salt

CONTAINS SOYBEAN AND WHEAT INGREDIENTS

Portion Sizes

Most of us tend to underestimate our food portion sizes. As a result, weighing and measuring your child's food to become more familiar with portion sizes and carb content is recommended. Tools can include measuring cups, measuring spoons, a food scale, food labels and a carbohydrate counting book.

It's All in Your Hand!

Another quick reference to determine portion sizes is to use your hand. The following are based on the average size of a woman's or adolescent's hand.

- Your fist is about the size of 1 cup
- Your palm is about the size of a 3 oz serving of meat or protein
- Your thumb is about
  - 1 ounce of cheese
  - 1 tablespoon of peanut butter or salad dressing
- Your thumb tip (the top joint of your thumb) is about one teaspoon

Or picture this…

• 1 ounce of meat or protein looks like 4 dice	• A medium piece of fruit is about the size of a tennis ball
• 1 ounce of cheese is about the size of a ping-pong ball	• A ½ cup grapes is equal to the size of a light bulb
• 1 tablespoon is the size of a walnut	• A medium potato is the size of a computer mouse
• 1 cup chopped fruit is the size of a baseball	

The more you practice weighing and measuring your child's food, the better you will be able to estimate portions and carbs when you are eating away from home.

Glycemic Index (GI) and Glycemic Load (GL)

Carb counting focuses on the amount of carb eaten, rather than the source of the carb. Some researchers suggest that carbohydrates affect blood glucose levels differently, depending on their source. Based on this idea, these researchers promote a meal-planning tool called the Glycemic

Index (GI). This nutrition approach, proposed for improving blood glucose control and/or weight loss, ranks foods according to their ability to raise blood glucose levels. For instance, the carb in a slice of 100% stone-ground whole wheat bread (low GI) may have less impact on your child's blood glucose level than a slice of processed white bread (high GI). It may be helpful to use the GI as an additional tool to understand differences in carb foods and how these differences impact your child's blood glucose levels.

Foods are compared to the speed at which glucose or white bread affects the blood glucose and, based on testing, given a GI number ranking. Glucose has a GI of 100. If the number is 70 or higher, the food is considered to have a high GI and have a faster affect on the blood glucose. If the number is 55 or lower, it has a low GI and has a slower affect on the blood glucose. Knowing the exact number is less important then knowing if it is a low, medium, or high GI food. In Table 7-8 are some examples of low, medium, and high GI foods.

- GI of 70 or more = High
- GI of 56 – 69 = Medium
- GI of 55 or less = Low

Table 7-8. Examples of Low, Medium, and High Glycemic Index (GI) Foods

Low GI Foods (GI is 55 or less)	Medium GI Foods (GI is 56-69)	High GI Foods (GI is 70 or more)
Whole grain breads	Rye bread	White bread
Bran cereals	Raisin Bran	Corn Chex
Green grapes	Fruit cocktail	Watermelon
Cooked barley	Canned sweet corn	Instant mashed potatoes
Milk	Soft drinks	Sports drinks

What else might affect the Glycemic Index of foods?

Many other factors will affect the GI of a food, listed below are some of the commons factors.

- **Protein and Fat.** These nutrients tend to slow the rate of stomach emptying and therefore the rate at which foods are digested in the small intestine. High-fat foods tend to have lower GI values than their low fat equivalents, but a lower GI food, like french fries, is not necessarily a healthy food choice. In general, low GI foods that are high in saturated or trans fats are unhealthy choices, despite having a low GI.

- **Fiber.** Refined grains, such as processed white bread, raise blood glucose more quickly than unrefined grains because fiber can act as a physical barrier to digestion. This decreases the rate at which carb is digested and therefore lowers the GI value. High fiber foods include whole grain breads and cereals, legumes, fresh fruits and vegetables.
- **Other Factors**
  - Food Factors
    - Food storage procedures
    - Cooking and processing methods
    - Ripeness
    - Acidity of the food
  - Human Factors
    - The rate at which you digest and absorb food
    - Your body weight
    - Pre-meal blood glucose level
    - Activity level
    - Time at which meals are eaten and foods eaten at a previous meal

What is Glycemic Load (GL)?

It is important to know the immediate effect that carb foods will have on blood glucose levels (GI) but for a more complete picture, we need to know the extent to which blood glucose rises and remains high. The Glycemic Load (GL) is the result of combining these 2 factors and will help determine the level a certain portion of a food will raise blood glucose levels. Calculating the GL takes the GI into account; we are provided with an estimate of both quality of carb (GI) and the quantity of carb (GL).

To calculate the Glycemic Load, multiply the GI value of a food by the amount of carbohydrate per serving and divide the result by 100: GL = (GI x carb grams/serving)/100. If the GL is greater than 20 it is considered to have a high GL and if less than 10 to have a low GL.

- GL of 20 or more = High
- GL of 11-19 = Medium
- GL of 10 or less = Low

For example, carrots have a GI of 92 and you may have been tempted to eliminate them from your child's meal plan, but common sense should tell you that carrots are a vegetable and provide nutrients and fiber. By calculating the GL, you can determine what portion size of carrots may work best for your child. The Glycemic Load (GL) takes the GI value divided by 100 then multiplied by the actual number of carbohydrates in a serving.

For 1/2 cup carrots (GI 92 x 4 g carb)/100 = GL 3.7 or 4 (Low)
For 2 cups carrots (GI 92 x 16 g carb)/100 = GL 15 (Medium)

For 1/2 cup pasta cooked (GI 64 x 20 g carb)/100 = GL 12.8 (Medium)
For 1 cup pasta cooked (GI 64 x 40 g carb)/100 = GL 25.6 (High)

For 1 cup watermelon (GI 72 x 12 g carb)/100 = GL 8.6 or 9 (Medium)
For 3 cups watermelon (GI 72 x 36 g carb)/100 = GL 26 (High)

In general the Glycemic Load is high when foods with a high Glycemic Index are eaten in large quantities. Therefore, you can reduce the GL by limiting foods that have a high GI or, when your child wants them, have smaller portions and/or adjust the insulin delivery. For example, if there are some meals that are enjoyed by the entire family but that always make your child's blood glucose high and you suspect it due to a high GL, delivering the insulin 20-30 minutes ahead of time and/or adding some additional insulin could help manage the blood glucose peak.

Special Dietary Considerations

Vegetarian

A vegetarian is someone who does not eat meat, fish or poultry. A vegetarian diet emphasizes whole grain foods, legumes, fruits, vegetables, nuts, and seeds. There are different types of vegetarian diets:

- **Semi-vegetarian:** excludes red meats, but occasionally eats fish or poultry and dairy products. Semi-vegetarians are often people who are making the transition to a vegetarian diet.
- **Lacto-ovo vegetarian:** excludes meat, fish, and poultry but includes milk, yogurt, cheese, and eggs.
- **Lacto-vegetarian:** excludes meat, fish, poultry, and eggs but includes milk and other dairy foods.
- **Pescetarians:** excludes meat or poultry but includes fish.
- **Vegan:** excludes *all* animal products (meat, fish, poultry, eggs, and dairy foods). A vegan eats only plant-based foods.

A well-planned vegetarian diet can be healthful and nutritionally adequate. Keep in mind that the more restricted the diet, the greater the chance of a nutritional deficiency. Vegetarian diets can provide an adequate amount of protein as long as your child eats a variety of foods and consumes enough calories to stay healthy. Protein is made up of amino acids, 9 of which are called essential amino acids. Animal foods contain all of the essential amino acids, whereas plant foods are missing 1 or 2. However, if your child eats a variety of plant foods, he or she will get all 9 essential amino acids.

If your child decides to become a vegetarian, it is recommended he or she visit with the dietitian to review his or her eating and make sure the chosen meal plan is adequate and nutritionally sound.

Celiac Disease and a Gluten-Free Diet

Celiac disease is an autoimmune disease that affects 6-14% of individuals with type 1 diabetes. Diagnosis is often difficult because symptoms are frequently minor or unusual and may even be nonexistent. If your healthcare provider suspects your child has celiac disease, she may order blood tests to measure the levels of antibodies to gluten. If the test comes back positive, your child will be referred to gastroenterologists for evaluation and may need a biopsy of his small intestine. Diagnosis is verified once improvement is seen when all gluten is removed from the diet and symptoms resolve.

Some of the signs and symptoms of celiac disease are as follows:

- Abdominal distention
- Abdominal pain
- Anemia
- Anorexia (poor appetite)
- Bloating
- Bone pain
- Constipation
- Cramping
- Dental hypoplasia (enamel missing on teeth)
- Dermatitis herpetiformis (rash)
- Diarrhea
- Failure to grow (children)
- Fatigue (tired, no energy)
- Folate deficiency
- Foul smelling stools
- Inability to concentrate
- Infertility in women
- Irritability
- Iron deficiency anemia
- Muscle cramps
- Osteopenia and osteoporosis (bone loss)
- Short stature
- Sleep disturbance
- Weakness
- Weight loss
- Vomiting

Treatment for celiac disease is the gluten-free diet, which avoids all sources of wheat, barley, and rye. Meeting with a dietitian who is familiar with celiac disease and diabetes can provide you accurate information and help you transition to the gluten-free diet as smoothly as possible.

Lactose Intolerance

Lactose is a sugar naturally present in milk and milk products, such as yogurt, cheese, and ice cream. In order to digest lactose, we have an enzyme in the intestine called lactase that breaks down lactose. People who do not make enough lactase cannot digest lactose. The inability to digest lactose is called lactose intolerance. Lactose intolerance is *not* the same as a milk allergy. Eating foods that contain lactose is not harmful if your child has lactose intolerance, but he or she may experience unpleasant symptoms. Symptoms can include nausea, abdominal cramps, bloating, gas, and diarrhea.

Lactose intolerance is very common in adults. Certain ethnic populations are affected more than others. Individuals are more likely to develop lactose intolerance if they are of African, Asian, Mexican, Mediterranean, or Jewish decent. Lactose intolerance increases as people age and is less common in young children. Primary lactose intolerance is genetic and is the most common type. Secondary (acquired) lactose intolerance may occur if the lining of the small intestine is damaged (from an illness, antibiotic use or celiac disease). Secondary lactose intolerance is usually temporary and will usually resolve.

Cholesterol and Children

According to the American Heart Association, elevated cholesterol levels early in life play a role in developing heart disease as an adult. Children with diabetes will be screened for cholesterol on a regular basis according to the American Diabetes Association (ADA) guidelines, especially if there is family history of high cholesterol and lipids. If your child's cholesterol is a concern, or you have a family history of high cholesterol, a change in nutrition habits can help lower cholesterol levels for most children and adolescents. The different types of lipids are listed below:

- **Total Cholesterol** is the total amount of cholesterol in your blood. It includes cholesterol made from your liver and sometimes

Table 7-9. Recommended Cholesterol Levels for Youth Aged 2-19

	Total Cholesterol	LDL Cholesterol	HDL Cholesterol	Triglycerides
Acceptable	Less than 170	Less than 110	Greater than 35	Less than 150
Borderline	170–199	110–129		
High	Greater than 200	Greater than 130		

Adapted from the National Cholesterol Education Program (NCEP) Guidelines

cholesterol from foods you eat. Your body uses cholesterol to make bile and hormones.

- **LDL Cholesterol** is considered the bad cholesterol because it carries fat towards the heart.
- **HDL Cholesterol** is considered the good cholesterol because it carries fat away from the heart.
- **Triglycerides** are the type of fat you burn for energy and store as body fat. High levels can increase your risk for heart disease.

Eating less fat and changing the type of fat eaten are heart-healthy choices for the entire family. Throughout this chapter and in practice, you will see that general healthy eating practices incorporate heart health. Here are some additional tips specific to lowering the unhealthy fats in your family's meal plan:

- Choose skim or 1% milk rather than 2% or whole milk (for children over the age of 2 years)
- For protein, eat poultry, fish, nuts, beans, soy, and leaner cuts of red meats. The leanest beef cuts usually include sirloin, chuck, loin, and round. Choose "choice" or "select" grades rather than "prime." Select lean or extra lean ground meats. Lean pork cuts include tenderloin or loin chops. The leanest lamb cuts come from the leg, arm, and loin.
- Use a "light," "trans fats free" tub margarine with plant stanols, rather than stick margarine or butter
- Bake, broil, grill, or steam foods instead of frying
- Cook with a monounsaturated fat, such as olive or canola oil, in moderation
- Add nuts to a salad or with fruit for a snack

- Limit processed snack foods like cookies and chips
- Eat "old fashioned" or "steel cut" oatmeal, oatmeal bread, beans, fruits, and vegetables for added soluble fiber
- Try eating fish at least 2-3 times a week, especially those types that are rich in omega-3 fats like salmon, trout, mackerel, halibut, and tuna

If your child's lipids are elevated, meeting with the RD will help you make additional non-pharmacological recommendations specific to your child's age, current dietary intake and daily activities.

Weight Management

Today it is estimated that 1 out of every 3 American children are overweight or obese. Children with diabetes are not immune to this national trend. Along with your pediatrician, your diabetes healthcare team will follow your child's growth very closely. If you, or the team, are concerned about your child's growth, it is suggested you visit with a pediatric dietitian to provide age-appropriate guidelines that best fit your child's individual needs. Many of the topics discussed in this chapter will help you provide a healthy nutrition foundation and eating behaviors that your child will carry throughout life.

References and Resources

Wheeler ML, Daly A, Evert A, Franz MJ, Geil P, Holzmeister LA, Kulkarmi K, Loghmani E, Ross TA, Woolf P. Choose your foods; exchange list for diabetes, sixth edition, 2008: description and guidelines for use. *J Am Diet Association*. 2008; 108:883-888.

U.S. Department of Health and Human Services and U.S. Department of Agriculture. Dietary Guidelines for Americans, 2005. 6th Edition, Washington, DC: U.S. Government Printing Office, January 2005.

United States Department of Agriculture, Center for Nutrition Policy and Promotion. MyPyramid for kids. MyPyramid.gov Website. 2009. Available at: http://mypyramid.gov/kids/index.html. Accessed April 6, 2009.

Adapted from Lowenberg, ME. Development of food patterns in young children. In: *Nutrition and Infancy and Childhood.* 5th ed. St Louis, MO: Mosby-Year Book; 1993:168-169.

Adapted from American Academy of Pediatrics, Committee on Nutrition. *Pediatric Nutrition Handbook.* 5th ed. Elk Grove Village, IL: American Academy of Pediatrics; 2004:128.

Institute of Medicine of the National Academies. *Dietary Reference Intakes for Energy, Carbohydrate, Fiber, Fat, Fatty Acids, Cholesterol, Protein, and Amino Acids (Macronutrients).* Washington, DC: National Academies Press, 2006.

Institute of Medicine of the National Academies. *Dietary Reference Intakes for Calcium, Phosphorus, Magnesium, Vitamin D, and Fluoride.* Washington, DC: National Academies Press, 1997.

Web sites:

- American Dietetic Association: www.eatright.org
- CalorieKing: www.calorieking.com/ —You can download a CalorieKing and Joslin Diabetes Center tool bar to your computer and have quick easy access to both sites on your internet browser
- Glycemic Index Information: www.glycemicindex.com
- United States Department of Agriculture, MyPyramid: www.mypyramid.gov

8

Physical Activity and Diabetes Management

Physical activity promotes health for children living with or without diabetes. Exercise contributes to improved quality of life, improved self-esteem, muscle development, team camaraderie, weight control, and it is fun!

The U.S. Department of Health and Human Services recommends that children exercise at least 60 minutes daily. Exercise includes play, organized sports, games, or any physical activity. Figure 8-1 gives you a bit more detail with a web site for further information.

If physical activity is considered a punishment or a chore, most people young and old alike, will not stick with the physical activity program. If kids have fun doing physical activity, whether alone, with family or with friends, they are more likely to want to continue it. School or community sports, varsity or intramural, all provide great opportunities for children and teens. Team sports such as baseball, football, hockey, basketball, and soccer not only encourage physical activity, they also provide a way to

Figure 8–1. Physical Activity Guidelines for Americans

Physical Activity Guidelines for Americans: October 2008
U.S. Department of Health & Human Services

Children and Adolescents – One hour or more of moderate or vigorous aerobic physical activity a day, including vigorous intensity physical activity at least three days a week. Examples of moderate intensity aerobic activities include hiking, skateboarding, bicycle riding and brisk walking. Vigorous intensity aerobic activities include bicycle riding, jumping rope, running and sports such as soccer, basketball and ice or field hockey. Children and adolescents should incorporate muscle-strengthening activities, such as rope climbing, sit-ups, and tug-of war, three days a week. Bone-strengthening activities, such as jumping rope, running and skipping, are recommended three days a week.

For more information see: www.cdc.gov/physicalactivity/everyone/guidelines/children.html

learn team play and sportsmanship and provide opportunities to meet other youth and experience winning and losing. Lifelong activities such as running, walking, hiking, bike riding, golf, and tennis provide exercise and enjoyment at any age.

So what if it is raining or no one is available to play a pick-up game of basketball, or it is dark out and your child can't go out running? There are other options:

- Video and video game systems offer some great options to get moving.
  - Dance Dance Revolution or similar programs
  - Wii or similar programs
  - Cable: Turn to one of the family-friendly music video or music stations to dance the time away
- Local gym membership may be available and discounted with health insurance. Consider a membership to a local YMCA. There may be great community resources like parks, tennis courts and town pools. Pack up the kids for a family fun outing of swimming, basketball or roller skating, for example.
- Change activities with the season
  - Winter: Is there an ice rink around?
  - Spring: How about volunteering to do a community winter cleanup?
  - Summer: Is there a community pool in your town?
  - Fall: Why not go apple picking?

If you as parents do not like physical activity and prefer to sit on the couch, your children will likely be couch potatoes. Despite what your children say, they want to be like their parents; so if you exercise, your kids will too. The following section addresses the benefits of exercise for your child's overall health and his or her diabetes management. But remember—knowing is not enough, doing is absolutely necessary.

Physical Activity and Diabetes

In children, adolescents, and young adults with diabetes, physical activity improves insulin sensitivity, burns excess glucose in the blood stream, maintains body weight, and improves overall A1C, cholesterol levels, and self-image. Both planned (games, organized sports) and unplanned (play) physical activity are equally important. For children with diabetes, balancing exercise, food intake, and insulin is important to minimize fluctuations of blood glucose levels. Children should always be praised for participating in physical activity and only held back from participating if their blood glucose and ketone levels are not in a safe range. In this chapter we will discuss physical activity with diabetes, the types of activity (anaerobic versus aerobic), blood glucose monitoring, and adjustments for planned and unplanned activity. Exercise by a person with diabetes can result in low blood glucose, high blood glucose, or target blood glucose levels. Understanding the effects of exercise on blood glucose levels will result in blood glucose levels in the target range.

During exercise the body's muscle cells need more energy to work harder. To explain the physiology of what happens when your child with diabetes exercises, it helps to review what happens in persons without diabetes. In children without diabetes, the body reduces insulin release from the beta cells in the pancreas and increases counter-regulatory hormones (cortisol, adrenaline, growth hormone, and glucagon). These counter-regulatory hormones tell the liver to release glucose into the bloodstream by breaking down glycogen — the storage form of glucose. (In fact, a glucagon emergency kit works to raise blood glucose during a severe low by breaking down the liver's stored glycogen.) The glycogen breakdown

Table 8–1. Effects of Exercise on Blood Glucose Levels: Keeping Levels in the Target Range

↓ Low Blood Glucose	Blood Glucose in Target	↑ High Blood Glucose
Too little food to cover for prolonged exercise	Increased carbohydrate intake before, during, and/or after exercise	Too little insulin before, during, and after exercise
Too much basal or bolus insulin	Pre-exercise insulin adjustment	Short spurts of anaerobic exercise causing the release counter-regulatory hormones
Unplanned, intensive workout	Blood glucose monitoring before, during, and after exercise	Too many carbohydrates consumed during exercise

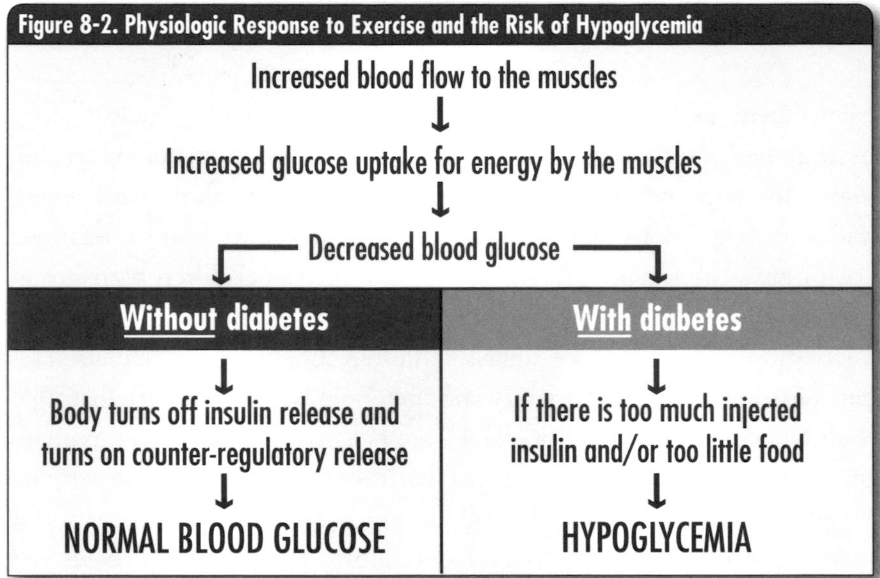

provides glucose (energy) to meet the increased glucose demands from the muscle cells during exercise. Therefore, the child without diabetes is able to avoid hypoglycemia (low blood glucose) with exercise. Hyperglycemia (high blood glucose) does not occur because the normally functioning beta cells in the pancreas release more insulin as soon as the blood glucose rises. Figure 8-2 depicts this process.

The muscles need insulin to use glucose. For children with diabetes, there must be enough insulin in the body for the muscles to work effectively and use the glucose for energy. Children cannot turn off or limit the insulin once it has been administered by syringe or insulin pump. Thus, it is necessary to ensure a constant source of glucose for the hard working muscles cells during physical activity. The counter-regulatory hormones, which are released during exercise in the person without diabetes, may not be released in the person with diabetes who has high insulin levels from injected or infused insulin.

Important: Remember that children with diabetes need a constant source of carbohydrates during and after exercise to ensure appropriate energy for the muscle cells and to prevent low blood glucose.

Considerations

Hypoglycemia

Hypoglycemia (low blood glucose) is the main risk factor when exercising with diabetes. In fact many hypoglycemic events in people living with diabetes are related to exercise. The longer the duration and the higher the intensity of physical activity, the more glucose is needed for the muscle cells to work. The way to prevent hypoglycemia with planned activity is to make adjustments to the insulin dose and/or eat more carbohydrate.

Guidelines for recommended blood glucose goals are shown in Table 8-2.

It is recommended that your child's blood glucose be checked before, during and after exercise and sometimes during the night following exercise. Ask your diabetes healthcare team for recommendations.

Table 8-2. Recommended Blood Glucose Goals

Age	Before Meals	Bedtime/Overnight	Before Exercise (Depending on Duration & Intensity)
Toddlers and Preschoolers (0–6)	100–180 mg/dL	110–200 mg/dL	150–200 mg/dL
School age (6–12)	90–180 mg/dL	100–180 mg/dL	150–200 mg/dL
Adolescents and Young adults (13–19)	90–130 mg/dL	90–150 mg/dL	150–200 mg/dL

Tips to Avoid Hypoglycemia Related to Physical Activity

- Children need approximately an extra 15 grams of carbohydrate for every 30 minutes of exercise.
- Adding fat and protein to meals and snacks helps avoid hypoglycemic reactions by providing a longer lasting form of energy than just carbohydrate.
- Adjusting insulin is another way to reduce the risk of hypoglycemia with exercise. Deciding whether to reduce the basal or bolus insulin dose is typically done when considering the timing, intensity, and duration of the activity. One often reduces insulin by 10–50%, again depending on the type of exercise.
- Avoid injecting insulin in the extremity that will be used during the exercise. Increased blood flow to the extremity during exercise may increase insulin's absorption, possibly leading to a low blood glucose.
- You may have heard the statement that exercise can drop your blood glucose level twice — once during the activity and once hours later. The second drop in blood glucose level is the so-called lag effect of exercise. This lag effect results from the muscles' need to replenish their stores of carbohydrates after exercise. Monitoring blood glucose and eating appropriate snacks and meals will help to minimize the possibility of a low blood glucose from the lag effect.

Children using insulin pumps and basal/bolus insulin plans can decrease the bolus of rapid-acting insulin for carbohydrates consumed before physical activity. This strategy works with planned activities rather than unplanned. To avoid hypoglycemia when wearing the insulin pump, the basal rate can also be decreased by 10–50%, depending on the duration and intensity of activity and past experiences. Work with your diabetes healthcare team to figure out the best plan to manage exercise for your child.

Hyperglycemia

Physical activity is important and fun for everyone. While activity is most often associated with low blood glucose levels, it may result in high blood glucose levels if there is not enough insulin available for the muscles to take up glucose for energy. Not having enough insulin in the body for a person with diabetes may lead to ketone formation and dehydration. It is important to avoid exercising whenever blood ketones exceed 0.6 mmol/L or urine ketones are small, moderate, or large, and whenever blood glucose levels are over 400 mg/dL (some healthcare professionals may say 300 mg/dL).

Hyperglycemia—Important Information

- Do not exercise
  - When blood glucose levels are greater than 400 mg/dL. Such a high blood glucose level indicates that there is not enough insulin to use for energy.
  - When blood ketones are above 0.6 mmol/l or urine ketones are small, moderate or large and the blood glucose is coming down.
- Take extra insulin, encourage fluids, and call your healthcare team for questions.

Insulin Guidelines for Physical Activity

Given that both insulin and physical activity can lower blood glucose, care needs to be given in managing insulin in relation to physical activity. Table 8-3 provides some tips on how to manage insulin. Speak with your healthcare team to determine the best options to manage your child's insulin during periods of exercise.

Table 8-3. Insulin Guidelines

Child with Insulin Pump	Child without Insulin Pump
• Use the temporary basal rate feature for 30-90 minutes before starting to exercise, during exercise and after. • Decrease the insulin to carbohydrate ratio (I:Carb) 1–4 hours prior to exercise. • If your child needs to disconnect from the insulin pump, check the blood glucose 30 minutes prior to exercise. Bolus half of the hourly basal before disconnecting to cover missed insulin when the pump is off during the activity. • Do not disconnect the pump for more than 2 hours. You can always reconnect briefly to give a bolus dose. • Check blood glucose levels 1 hour into exercise and correct blood glucose as needed. During exercise your child may have a higher target glucose like 150, 180, or even 200 mg/dL.	• For children using basal/bolus insulin therapy, cut the insulin to carb ratio (I:Carb) in half when eating meals or snacks up to 1–2 hours before exercising. • Make sure to have an extra 15 grams of carbohydrate for every 30 minutes of exercise. • To avoid the lag effect, make sure to have extra carbohydrates at bedtime, or if using I:Carb ratios, give less insulin for food. For example, instead of using a 1:10 g I:Carb ratio, use a 1:15 g I:Carb ratio. • For all day activities, consult with your diabetes team to decrease the intermediate or basal insulin the morning of or night prior to exercise and again decrease the insulin after the exercise. The intermediate or basal insulin might be decreased by 10–20%, for example.

Anaerobic verses Aerobic Activity

There are 2 distinct types of exercise, aerobic and anaerobic.

1. **Aerobic exercise** means that the work performed by the muscles uses oxygen when deriving energy from glucose. Aerobic means "with oxygen."
2. **Anaerobic exercise** means that the work performed by the muscles does not use oxygen when deriving energy from glucose. Anaerobic means "without oxygen." It refers to the initial phase of exercise, or to any short burst of intense exertion, in which the glycogen or sugar is consumed without oxygen; it is a far less efficient process.

Muscles need insulin in order to use glucose for energy, so if insulin isn't present, or when carbohydrates (glucose) are all used up, muscles convert to using fat for energy.

There are many kinds of aerobic exercise. Aerobic exercise usually includes fitness or fat-burn activities and cardio or endurance training. Aerobic exercise usually lasts for extended periods, and starts with a warm-up and ends with a cool-down. See Table 8-4 for a listing of many kinds of

Table 8-4. Examples of Aerobic and Anaerobic Activities

Aerobic Activity	Anaerobic Activity
Running	Weight lifting
Swimming (distance)	Swimming (sprint)
Hiking	Sports with bursts of energy (hockey, football, diving)
Cycling	Running (sprints)
Walking	
Skiing	

aerobic exercise. Anaerobic exercise usually includes strength training or weight training. Anaerobic exercise is usually intense activity that lasts for seconds to minutes at a time. Both sprints as well as weight lifting or resistance training are forms of anaerobic exercise. An exercise program should include both aerobic and anaerobic activities for maximal conditioning.

Aerobic and anaerobic activity can affect the blood glucose in different ways. Typically, aerobic exercise is a continuous activity, like running, swimming, and cycling. It is sometimes referred to as cardio exercise. With aerobic exercise, the blood glucose drops 20-60 minutes after the onset of activity. Anaerobic exercise, with its short bursts of activity, leads to surges of counter-regulatory hormones (adrenaline and glucagon, for example) that can cause the blood glucose to increase dramatically. While aerobic activities often lead to low glucose levels, it is anaerobic exercise that may initially raise the blood glucose level. However, both anaerobic and aerobic exercise can lead to low blood glucose levels, especially due to the lag effect.

Anaerobic and Aerobic Activity and the Lag Effect

Both aerobic and anaerobic exercise can result in the lag effect of exercise. The lag effect is when the blood glucose may drop several hours after exercise. The body is replacing the glycogen stores in the muscle.

Duration and Intensity

Duration and intensity of physical activity have a big effect on blood glucose levels. When exercising for longer than 30 minutes at a time, hypoglycemia and hyperglycemia are inevitable if the diabetes management plan is not altered. Short bursts of physical activity, like a 10-second sprint during a run, can help blood glucose levels from dropping. This is due to the release of the counter-regulatory hormones during that brief sprint (anaerobic activity). Organized sports, like soccer, require more planning because of the long duration and moderate to heavy intensity levels. Remember, work with your diabetes team when it comes to making insulin adjustments and/or increasing carbohydrate intake prior to, during, or after activity.

As physical activity causes dehydration, it is important to keep well hydrated during exercise. Consider a sports drink that provides some carbohydrates if your child gets thirsty during sports. By diluting the sports drink with water, he or she can drink often and get a small, steady amount of carbs during the activity.

Table 8-5 provides snack options for exercise.

Table 8-5. Snack Options for Exercise: Nutrition Bars, Drinks and Miscellaneous Snacks

Nutrition Bars					
Item	**Calories**	**Carbohydrates**	**Protein**	**Fat**	**Comments**
Power gel 1.4 oz	110 kcal	28 grams	0 grams	0 grams	Assorted Flavors
GU 32 grams	100 kcal	25 grams	0 grams	0 grams	Assorted Flavors
PowerBar 65 grams	230 kcal	45 grams	10 grams	2 grams	Assorted Flavors
PowerBar Harvest 65 grams	240 kcal	45 grams	7 grams	4 grams	Assorted Flavors
Cliff Bar 68 grams	240 kcal	46 grams	10 grams	4 grams	Organic; No High Fructose Corn Syrup; 5 grams of fiber
Balance 50 grams	190 kcal	22 grams	14 grams	6 grams	Assorted Flavors
Glucerna 40 grams	150 kcal	25 grams	6 grams	4 grams	Assorted Flavor
Luna Bar 48 grams	180 kcal	28 grams	10 grams	3.5 grams	Organic nutrient bar; No High Fructose Corn Syrup
Mojo Bar 45 grams	180 kcal	22 grams	10 grams	9 grams	Assorted Flavors Nuts & Pretzels
South Beach Bar 35 grams	140 kcal	15 grams	10 grams	5 grams	

<table>
<tr><th colspan="6">Drink Options</th></tr>
<tr><td>Item</td><td>Calories</td><td>Carbohydrates</td><td colspan="3">Comments</td></tr>
<tr><td>Gatorade
8 oz</td><td>50 kcal</td><td>14 grams</td><td colspan="3">Assorted Flavors</td></tr>
<tr><td>Accelerade
8 oz</td><td>80 kcal</td><td>15 grams</td><td colspan="3">Assorted Flavors</td></tr>
<tr><td>Powerade
8 oz</td><td>60 kcal</td><td>17 grams</td><td colspan="3">Mountain Blast</td></tr>
<tr><td>Trek
8 oz</td><td>70 kcal</td><td>16 grams</td><td colspan="3"></td></tr>
<tr><td>1% Milk
8 oz</td><td>110 kcal</td><td>13 grams</td><td colspan="3">To prevent delayed hypoglycemia post exercise 8 grams protein; 2.5 grams fat</td></tr>
<tr><th colspan="6">Miscellaneous Snacks</th></tr>
<tr><td>Item</td><td>Calories</td><td>Carbohydrates</td><td>Protein</td><td>Fat</td><td>Comments</td></tr>
<tr><td>Graham Crackers (3)</td><td>90 kcal</td><td>17 grams</td><td>1.5 grams</td><td>1.5 grams</td><td></td></tr>
<tr><td>Apple
Med. 5 oz</td><td>60 kcal</td><td>18 grams</td><td></td><td></td><td></td></tr>
<tr><td>Peanut Butter Nabs (4)</td><td>130 kcal</td><td>15 grams</td><td>3 grams</td><td>7 grams</td><td></td></tr>
<tr><td>Kellogg's Nutri grain
37 grams</td><td>140 kcal</td><td>27 grams</td><td>2 grams</td><td>3 grams</td><td>Assorted Flavors</td></tr>
<tr><td>Banana Med.
7-8" long</td><td>108 kcal</td><td>27 grams</td><td></td><td></td><td></td></tr>
</table>

Summary

By careful monitoring of blood glucose and adjusting the insulin doses and/or carbohydrate intake for physical activity, a child can enjoy the benefits of activity and avoid swings in blood glucose levels. Work with your diabetes healthcare team to help successfully manage diabetes with exercise and have fun. Just keep in mind the following:

Check List of Exercise Planning for Children with Diabetes

- ✓ Be sure that coaches, physical education teachers, and others in a leadership role know that your child has diabetes and understands the need to watch out for symptoms of hypoglycemia.
- ✓ Be sure that your child wears a medical ID noting the diagnosis of

diabetes. The ID may need to come off during the athletic event — this is not a problem, especially since the coaches, etc., are aware that your child has diabetes. Be sure to have a safe place to store the ID and help your child remember to put it back on after the athletic event.

- ✓ Bring your child's blood glucose meter, lancets, and strips so that he or she is able to check blood glucoses during the physical activity.
- ✓ If your child wears an insulin pump with a traditional infusion set (rather than a pod-type pump), be sure to have a safe storage place to keep the pump if he or she disconnects for sporting events and remember to reconnect the pump after the event. Bolus, as needed, before disconnecting, during the event, and upon reconnecting. And remember never, never disconnect more the 2 hours!
- ✓ Bring plenty of fluids for hydration, water or sports drinks, as well as snack foods and rapid acting carb snacks, like glucose tabs, to treat low blood glucose if and when it occurs.
- ✓ Remember to check blood glucose levels after the athletic event to monitor for possible lag effects of the exercise.
- ✓ Have fun!!!

References and Resources

Kollipara S, Warren-Boulton E. School *Nurse News*. 2004 May;21(3):12-6.

Sigal RJ, Kenny GP, Wasserman DH, Castaneda-Sceppa C. Physical activity/exercise and type 2 diabetes. *Diabetes Care*. 2004;27:2518–2539.

Tansey MJ, Tsalikian E, Beck RW, Mauras N, Buckingham BA, Weinzimer SA et al. The effects of aerobic exercise on glucose and counterregulatory hormone concentrations in children with type 1 diabetes. *Diabetes Care*. 2006; 29(1):20-25.

American Diabetes Association. Diabetes mellitus and exercise. *Diabetes Care*. 2002; 25(Supplement 1):S64-S68.

Galassetti PR, Iwanaga K, Crisostomo M, Zaldivar FP, Larson J, Pescatello A. Inflammatory cytokine, growth factor and counterregulatory responses to exercise in children with type 1 diabetes and healthy controls. *Pediatr Diabetes*. 2006; 7(1):16-24.

Web sites:

- Diabetes Exercise and Sports Association: www.diabetes-exercise.org
- Medical Identification Products: www.childrenwithdiabetes.com
- http://www.childrenwithdiabetes.com

9

Hypoglycemia

Hypoglycemia means low blood glucose and is sometimes called an insulin reaction or a low. It is a reversible, short-term complication that can affect any child treated with insulin. It is important that you and your child understand the causes, signs, and symptoms, and treatment of hypoglycemia. With this knowledge, you and your child will be able to better prevent and treat episodes of hypoglycemia.

For a child treated with insulin, hypoglycemia is defined as a blood glucose level less than 60 mg/dL. People who do not use insulin can have a blood glucose level below 60 mg/dL without any problems because their bodies are able to use other sources of energy, such as fat. Insulin not only lowers the blood glucose, but it also prevents the body from using fat for energy. Therefore, children treated with insulin *must* have enough glucose in order for the body to function normally.

Table 9-1 summarizes the causes, symptoms, and treatments of hypoglycemia — low blood glucose levels.

Signs and Symptoms of Hypoglycemia

Your child may feel and act differently if he or she becomes *hypoglycemic* (which means he or she is having an episode of hypoglycemia). Symptoms are ways a person *feels* while signs are changes someone else can see occurring in the person. The signs and symptoms usually become more severe as the blood glucose goes lower. It is very important that you, other caretakers (like grandparents, teachers, friends' parents) and your child know the various signs and symptoms that occur with hypoglycemia. This will allow you to act quickly to prevent a more severe reaction. Some common signs and symptoms of hypoglycemia are:

- Shaky
- Sweaty
- Hungry
- Dizzy or lightheaded
- Weakness
- Irritability
- Tiredness
- Headache
- Blurry or double vision
- Confusion

If your child has a hypoglycemic or low blood glucose event, you should talk about the symptoms that your child experienced and remember the signs that you noticed. This information will allow you both to identify and manage future episodes of hypoglycemia. When a child is very

Table 9-1. Hypoglycemia: Causes, Symptoms, and What to Do

Hypoglycemia Causes	Symptoms	What to Do
• Too much insulin • Insufficient food (carbohydrate) • Physical activity (especially long duration, high intensity, or unplanned) • Illness (especially in setting of vomiting) • Medications • Pregnancy (1st trimester) • Alcohol use	• Shaky • Sweaty • Hungry • Dizzy or lightheaded • Weakness • Irritability • Tiredness • Headache • Blurry or double vision • Confusion	• Always carry hypoglycemia treatment for your child (see Table 9-2) • Understand your child's signs and symptoms of hypoglycemia and always check his or her blood glucose level if your child feels or appears to be low • Take time to calculate insulin doses • Make sure enough carbohydrate is eaten after insulin is given; if your child is very young or sick, your provider may discuss alternatives to giving the entire insulin dose before meals and/or setting a temporary basal rate for insulin pump users • Reduce insulin or increase carbohydrate intake before exercise or drinking alcohol • Frequent blood glucose monitoring, especially if your child has hypoglycemic unawareness, does not feel well or is in a situation that places him or her at risk for hypoglycemia (i.e., exercise) • During an illness, if your child is unable to eat or is vomiting, call your healthcare team to discuss insulin adjustments and blood glucose management • Discuss unexplained hypoglycemia with your healthcare team

young, it is common that he or she will not be able to recognize and tell you about these symptoms — what is generally called feeling low. This is called *hypoglycemia unawareness.*

Hypoglycemic unawareness is when a child does not have any symptoms related to a low blood glucose level. Children who do not feel different when the blood glucose is low are at higher risk for a severe hypoglycemic reaction; this is most common among young children who take insulin. During this time, you cannot rely on your child to tell you that he or she is feeling low. You must rely on the signs that you recognize and blood glucose monitoring results to identify hypoglycemia.

Consequences of Hypoglycemia

Seizures and loss of consciousness are the most serious consequences of hypoglycemia and are frequently referred to as severe reactions. Although these consequences are certainly enough reason to avoid hypoglycemia, there are also indirect consequences of hypoglycemia which are equally serious. If your child becomes confused or disoriented from hypoglycemia, there is an increased risk of injury from accidents and falls. For a teenager, this includes driving accidents, which can place your child and others at risk. Performance at school and/or work can decline when someone becomes hypoglycemic.

Emotional and psychological reactions following a hypoglycemic episode can be stressful and complicate diabetes management. This often occurs following a severe reaction or an incident that occurred in public that was embarrassing to the child. *Fear of hypoglycemia* is a psychological response by a child or caregiver to a hypoglycemic event, such as seizure or loss of consciousness. The emotional distress causes the child or caregiver to allow blood glucose values to stay high (often times well above the recommended range) in order to reduce the risk of hypoglycemia in the future. Although the child or parent recognizes the risk of complications associated with hyperglycemia, they have a difficult time readjusting after the hypoglycemic event.

Causes of Hypoglycemia

So what causes hypoglycemia? As you know, insulin lowers blood glucose levels. If too much insulin is given, your child is at risk for developing hypoglycemia. The first types of insulin used to treat diabetes successfully lowered blood glucose, but not in the same way the body naturally uses insulin. Blood glucose and insulin levels did not rise and fall together. Fortunately, the rapid-acting analogues now in use allow you and your child to have blood glucose and insulin levels that more closely rise and fall together. Studies have shown that these rapid-acting analogues reduce the risk of hypoglycemia.

There are situations when your child is at risk for hypoglycemia even if the correct amount of insulin is given at the right time. The following are situations that can cause hypoglycemia:

- Too much insulin
- Insufficient food (carbohydrate)
- Physical activity (especially long duration, high intensity, or unplanned)
- Illness (especially in setting of vomiting)
- Medications
- Pregnancy (1st trimester)
- Alcohol use

During exercise, your child's body (especially those active muscles!) requires more energy than normal. This energy is glucose. Therefore, exercise can lower your child's blood glucose. The amount the blood glucose falls is usually related to *how long* and *how demanding* your child's activity is. Regular physical activity is very important to the health and happiness of your child. You might expect the blood glucose to fall during exercise when the body is most active. Studies have shown that the fall in blood glucose can occur *hours* after your child is finished exercising. See Chapter 8: Physical Activity and Diabetes Management for more information on exercise.

Illness is another situation that increases the risk of hypoglycemia. When your child is sick, he or she may not be willing or able to eat as much as usual. This is particularly true during vomiting illnesses such as the stomach flu. Despite this, insulin doses may increase during illness to prevent ketone formation. If the blood glucose levels are already low because of limited eating or vomiting, this additional insulin can lead to hypoglycemia. Checking blood glucose levels frequently is necessary during any type of illness.

There are other situations which may increase the risk of hypoglycemia, such as other medications which can lower blood glucose values. Some medications can cause hypoglycemia in combination with insulin therapy. It is important that you ask your healthcare provider or pharmacist if medications your child uses can lower — or raise — your child's blood glucose values.

Alcohol can lower blood glucose values. If people with type 1 diabetes are not cautious while drinking alcoholic beverages, they are at high risk for severe hypoglycemic reactions. Why? The liver stores unused carbohydrates after meals and can make glucose from it for your body. This allows the liver to provide one's body energy and prevent hunger between meals. Alcohol can prevent the liver from releasing glucose even if the blood glucose is falling or already low. As more alcohol is consumed, the risk of severe hypoglycemia increases. Although alcoholic drinks contain carbohydrates and can raise the blood glucose in the short-term, it is important to think about preventing hypoglycemia when consuming alcohol.

Preventing and Treating Hypoglycemia

Once you recognize the possible causes and consequences of hypoglycemia, it is important to realize that there are many ways to prevent and, if necessary, treat hypoglycemia. This is especially true for severe hypoglycemia. While some of these steps are very simple, they are all important for you and those who care for your child to understand. Let's start with prevention.

The following are *key steps to preventing hypoglycemia:*

- Always carry hypoglycemia treatment for your child (see Table 9-2).

- Understand your child's signs and symptoms of hypoglycemia and *always* check his or her blood glucose level if your child feels or appears to be low.
- Take time to calculate insulin doses.
- Make sure enough carbohydrate is eaten after insulin is given; if your child is very young or sick, your provider may discuss alternatives to giving the entire insulin dose before meals and/or setting a temporary basal rate for insulin pump users.
- Reduce insulin or increase carbohydrate intake before exercise or drinking alcohol.
- Frequent blood glucose monitoring, especially if your child has hypoglycemic unawareness, does not feel well or is in a situation that places him or her at risk for hypoglycemia (*i.e.*, exercise).
- During an illness, if your child is unable to eat or is vomiting, call your healthcare team to discuss insulin adjustments and blood glucose management.
- Discuss unexplained hypoglycemia with your healthcare team.

While it is important to know how to prevent hypoglycemia, all children who take insulin occasionally will have episodes of hypoglycemia. It is critical that you know how to treat hypoglycemia. Since it is important to prevent hypoglycemia, treatment should be given for blood glucose readings less than 80 mg/dL. The treatment depends on the blood glucose reading and your child's symptoms. Mild hypoglycemia occurs when the blood glucose value is below 80 mg/dL whether or not your child has symptoms. Severe hypoglycemia occurs when your child, when old enough, cannot treat the hypoglycemia without someone else's help due to severe confusion, loss of consciousness, or seizure. The risk of severe hypoglycemia increases when the blood glucose reading is below 40 mg/dL.

If there is a concern for hypoglycemia, your child should immediately stop what he or she is doing. For example, your child should stop taking a test at school, playing in a sporting event, or pull over into the emergency lane while driving. *It is critical to address a possible low blood glucose as soon as possible*. It is important to confirm your child's blood glucose with a finger stick blood glucose check when he or she feels low. A blood glucose meter should always be with your child. If you are in a situation where you suspect your child is hypoglycemic but are unable to check your child's blood glucose, you should assume that he or she is hypoglycemic and treat without checking the blood glucose value.

Treating Mild Hypoglycemia

For mild hypoglycemia, use the 15-15 rule. The 15-15 rule states that:

- **15 grams** of fast-acting carbohydrate should be eaten followed
- **15 minutes** later with a blood glucose recheck
  - If the blood glucose remains less than 80 mg/dL after 15 minutes, an additional 15 grams of carbohydrate should be given.
  - This can be repeated until the blood glucose level rises above 80 mg/dL. You should consider rechecking the blood glucose more frequently after this, but do not give additional carbohydrates if the level is above 80 mg/dL.
  - It is also important to remember that *the symptoms of hypoglycemia can take longer to recover from than the actual blood glucose value*. If you can check your child's blood glucose, do not continue treating symptoms without knowing your child's blood glucose reading — this could lead to over treatment and result in high blood glucose (hyperglycemia).

Table 9-2. Hypoglycemia Treatment: Sources and Appropriate Quantities of Fast-Acting Carbohydrate

Age	5 years or younger	6 to 10 years	Over 10 years
Amount required	5–10 grams carb	10–15 grams carb	15–20 grams carb
Glucose tablets	1–2 tablets	2–3 tablets	3–4 tablets
Insta-glucose	⅓–½ tube	½–⅔ tube	⅔–1 tube
Regular soda	2–3 ounces	4–5 ounces	5–6 ounces
Juice (apple, orange)	¼–½ cup	½–¾ cup	¾–1 cup
Cake icing	2 teaspoons	3 teaspoons	4–5 teaspoons
Honey or syrup	2 teaspoons	3 teaspoons	4–5 teaspoons
Raisins	1 tablespoon	1½–2 tablespoons	2½ tablespoons

Appropriate hypoglycemic treatments with age-related doses are listed in Table 9-2.

When treating hypoglycemia, do not use foods that are high in fat or protein, like chocolate. Fat and protein can delay the rise in blood glucose.

Treating Severe Hypoglycemia

Severe hypoglycemia is defined as a low blood glucose level that requires someone else's assistance to treat. It is not defined by a specific blood glucose value, but the risk increases as the blood glucose goes lower. Severe hypoglycemia is a medical emergency and can result in seizure or loss of consciousness. If your child is unconscious or having a seizure, never try to feed her fast-acting carbohydrate — she could choke on the food or drink. Glucagon is the medical treatment for severe hypoglycemia.

Once the glucagon is injected, glucose stored in the liver enters the bloodstream. This results in a rapid rise in blood glucose. The blood glucose should rise 50-75 mg/dL within 15-20 minutes. Typically, this rise will terminate the severe reaction. If your child does not have enough glucose stored in the liver, *glucagon may not work.* If your child does not stop seizing or wake up within 1-2 minutes after the glucagon injection, call 911.

WARNING: If your child does not stop seizing or wake up after the glucagon, call 911.

Your healthcare team will instruct you on how to prepare and administer glucagon. Figure 9-1 depicts the process.

Glucagon Dose

The dose of glucagon is based on your child's weight:

- 0.3 mg (0.3 mL = 30 units) for children less than 25 pounds
- 0.5 mg (0.5 mL = 50 units) for children between 25-50 pounds
- 1.0 mg (1.0 mL = 100 units) for children over 50 pounds

For severe hypoglycemia, glucagon is typically *injected into muscle* with the

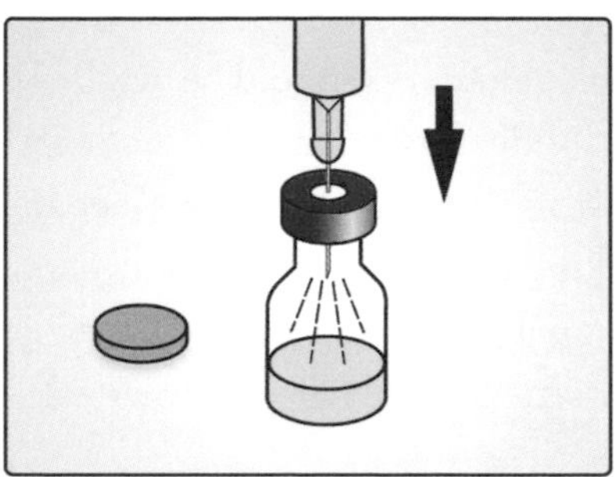

Push the orange plastic cap off the vial. Pull the needle cover off the syringe, and insert the needle through the rubber disc of the vial. Inject all the liquid from the syringe into the vial.

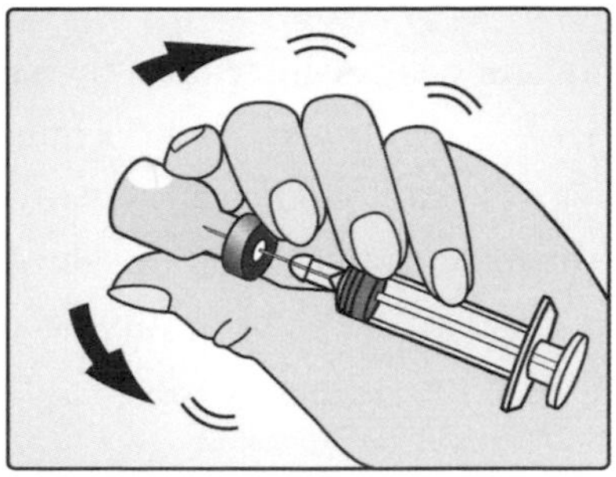

Without withdrawing the syringe and needle, gently shake the vial until the glucagon is completely dissolved and the solution is clear.

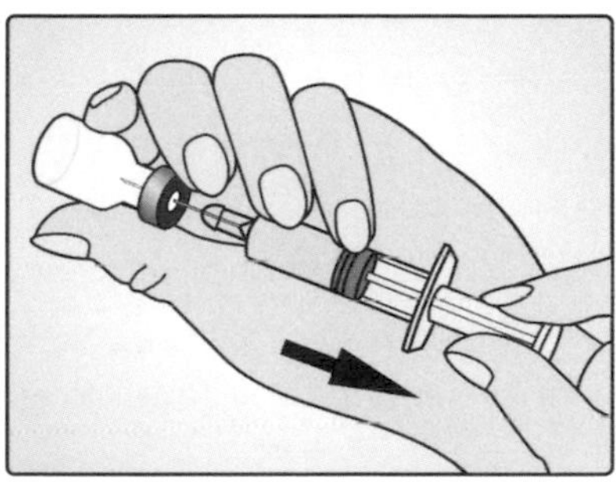

Ensure that the plunger is completely depressed. Withdraw all of the solution back into the syringe. Be careful that the plunger is not pulled out of the syringe.

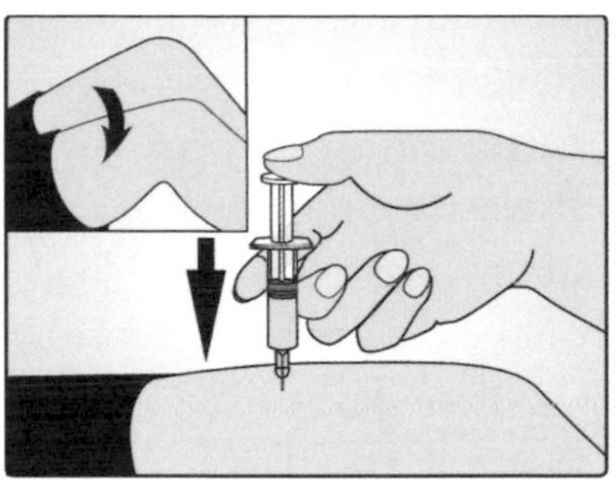

The solution is used for injection. Ensure there is no air remaining in the syringe before giving the injection.

FIGURE 9-1. Preparing Glucagon

needle provided in the emergency kit. Your healthcare team may discuss administering glucagon with an insulin syringe.

Once you have injected glucagon, remember:

- Keep your child on his side; glucagon can cause vomiting
- Do not leave your child if at all possible
- Call 911 if necessary
- Feed your child as soon as she is awake and able to eat
- If your child has not revived in 15 minutes, give another shot of glucagon

Glucagon emergency kits should always be available at home and while traveling. You should discuss keeping additional glucagon kits elsewhere with your healthcare team. When possible, glucagon should be available at school — ideally with a school nurse. Individual state laws may dictate who can give your child glucagon, particularly in the school setting. Keep track of the expiration date on the glucagon kits. Before throwing away expired kits, use them to practice mixing and drawing up glucagon — *never* inject glucagon into someone who is not experiencing severe hypoglycemia.

Mini-Dose Glucagon

There are situations when your child may be awake and have hypoglycemia, but he or she may not be willing or able to eat. The 2 most common situations are hypoglycemia in infants or very young children, and vomiting illnesses. In the past, children would often go to the Emergency Room to receive intravenous fluids containing dextrose (a type of glucose). As an alternative, you can give your child a small dose of glucagon using an insulin syringe to raise the blood glucose. This is called mini-dose glucagon and should be reviewed with your healthcare team.

The mini-dose of glucagon is based on your child's *age* not weight. Doses are described in Table 9-3.

The glucagon is mixed using the needle in the kit, but *drawn up using an insulin syringe*. The mini-glucagon dose should raise the blood glucose within 15-20 minutes. If blood glucose rises, but not enough, the mini-dose of glucagon can be repeated. Often times, the rise is temporary. You must continue to monitor your child's blood glucose to make sure it remains in range. If your child does not have enough glucose stored in the liver, glucagon will not work. You should not try to repeat doses of glucagon if the initial attempt does not raise the blood glucose.

If mini-dose glucagon does not raise the blood glucose, your child should be taken to a local Emergency Department for intravenous fluids containing glucose. If you are concerned about your child's health and safety, or simply getting to a local hospital, call 911.

Table 9-3. Mini-Dose Glucagon Based on Age

Age	Dose
Children 2 years or younger	2 units
Children 3–14 years	1 unit for every year of life (e.g., 5 units for 5-year old)
Children 15 years or older	15 units

Summary

Hypoglycemia is a risk for all people with type 1 diabetes. Hypoglycemia is in fact the result of the treatment for diabetes (insulin) not diabetes itself. Anyone caring for your child should understand how to recognize and treat mild to severe hypoglycemia. Always keep fast-acting carbs with your child. A glucagon emergency kit should always be available at home and while traveling; ideally, glucagon should be kept at school with a trained professional. Severe hypoglycemia is a medical emergency; if you are worried about the health and safety of your child, call 911.

References and Resources

Haymond MW, Schreiner B. Mini-dose glucagon rescue for hypoglycemia in children with type 1 diabetes. *Diabetes Care*. 2001;24(4):643-645.

Evert AB. Managing hypoglycemia in the school setting. School Nurse News 2005; 22(5):16-20.

Hasan KS, Kabbani M. Mini-dose glucagon is effective at diabetes camp. *J Pediatr*. 2004; 144(6):834.

Web sites:

- Eli Lilly Glucagon Emergency Kit: www.humalog.com
- Novo Nordisk GlucaGen HypoKit: www.novonordiskcare.com
- Children with Diabetes: Robin - The Importance of Having a Glucagon Emergency Kit on Hand at All Times: www.childrenwithdiabetes.com

10

Hyperglycemia and Insulin Adjustments

Hyperglycemia is the medical term for high blood glucose. Whether at diagnosis or with day-to-day diabetes self management, the causes, symptoms, and treatments of high blood glucoses are the same. Table 10.1 summarizes the causes, symptoms, and treatments of high blood glucose levels.

Knowing your child's target blood glucose range helps you to know if a blood glucose is low, in-range, or high. Many factors will be considered by your healthcare team to determine your child's individual goals for blood glucose targets. Factors include:

- Chronological age
- Duration of diabetes
- Available family and school supports
- Child temperament and cooperation with the diabetes management plan
- Child's cognitive ability to participate in assisting in self-management of diabetes
- Recognition of the symptoms of high and/or low blood glucose levels

Taking all of these factors into consideration, the treatment for hyperglycemia varies by factors such as age, time of day, and/or the cause of the hyperglycemia. For example, if your child is 6, you would not aim for as tight glycemic control as if your child were 16. The blood glucose target range determines how and when you treat a high blood glucose level. If it is your child's bedtime, you would treat with a more conservative dose of

Table 10-1. Hyperglycemia: Causes, Symptoms, and Treatments

Hyperglycemia Causes	Symptoms	Treatments
• illness/infection • too little insulin • insulin has lost potency (expired usage or shelf life) • insulin storage or duration problems • timing of insulin doses • air bubbles • too much food • not enough exercise • change in schedule or activity • increased insulin requirements with growth • stresses	• thirst • increased urination (trouble toilet training or bedwetting) • blurred vision • mood swings • hunger (sometimes no hunger at all) • weight loss or poor weight gain • nausea and/or vomiting	• call the healthcare team • give extra insulin supplements using rapid- or fast-acting insulin boosters • adjust the dose of insulin

insulin to avert potential nighttime hypoglycemia. Safety is always the first consideration.

A high blood glucose number should never be considered bad nor should a child be made to feel badly about this number. It is easy to feel that you or your child is to blame for the number and feel like a failure. Frustration can occur. But remember, all information is good information; it can be used to measure insulin dose effectiveness and safety. Neither you nor your child should feel discouraged about out-of-range numbers, especially when you consider that there are a number of causes for elevated blood glucose values, some of which you have no control over. What is important is to use the information to problem solve to decrease the frequency and duration of high blood glucose levels.

Causes of Hyperglycemia

Making diabetes and its related tasks a family affair means that the family shares in working together to manage diabetes. Managing diabetes is hard work! The list of causes for high glucose values is long. High blood glucose levels can be unique to the individual or the situation. Insulin, insulin delivery devices, injection sites, food, activity levels, hormones, illness and infection, medication, and hypoglycemia can all be related to elevations in blood glucose levels. The following section provides you with more information on how this occurs. Though some of the information also appears in specific chapters of the book, it bears repeating in this chapter in the context of finding out why your child may be having episodes of hyperglycemia.

Insulin and Hyperglycemia

Important considerations of hyperglycemia resulting from an error in insulin dose may be related to:

- Expired insulin
- Insulin storage or duration problems
- Timing of insulin doses
- Air bubbles

Insulin Delivery Devices and Hyperglycemia

Important considerations of hyperglycemia resulting from an error in the delivery of insulin from an insulin delivery device may be related to:

- Insulin syringe: Look carefully at the insulin syringe to ensure that you understand how to interpret the lines on the syringe.
- Needle length: Does the syringe have a standard or short needle on it? Short needles may not deposit the insulin far enough beneath the skin in heavier youth. Signs of this might be complaints of stinging with injections, insulin leakage or a raised welt at the injection site.
- Priming: If using an insulin pen, there needs to be a priming of the needle tip prior to dialing an insulin dose. The priming dose fills the tip of the pen needle to ensure your child is receiving the entire dose of insulin. This involves dialing 2 units and then depressing the plunger to express those 2 units into a sink or wastebasket. Remember, once insulin has been injected, slowly count to 5 to ensure that the dose has been fully delivered before withdrawing the needle.

Rotation of Sites

One of the most important roles a parent can play in insulin administration involves support in site selection. We all get into a routine of doing what is easiest and most comfortable, and that includes injection site use. Developing a method of ensuring that the injection sites are well rotated will help minimize hypertrophy, an area of exaggerated fat growth under the skin that occurs when insulin is repeatedly injected into the same site. Hypertrophy, on inspection, looks like a puffy area of tissue or feels like a lump or bump at the injection site. Insulin injected into a site with hypertrophy does not work well or consistently. In addition, cosmetically, it causes concern for many youth, especially if noticeable on areas like the arms or thighs if not covered by clothing. When this occurs, avoiding the site will allow the tissue to return to normal. For additional information on hypertrophy see Chapter 4: Insulin.

Site Absorption Rates

Insulin can be absorbed from different sites at varying rates. Insulin is absorbed fastest from the abdomen, followed by the arm, thigh, and slowest from the buttocks. These differences may not serve to alter blood glucose levels significantly, but many parents use this concept for making a purposeful decision about site selection based on blood glucose level; the more elevated the blood glucose level, the more likely the injection is in the abdomen. As a parent and another set of eyes looking at injection sites, you want to be observant of tissue appearance and texture. Thickened, puffy sites will not absorb insulin in a predictable manner and will lead to erratic and elevated blood glucose levels.

Insulin Leakage

Hypertrophied injection sites have a greater tendency for insulin leakage. If insulin is leaking from the injection site, the blood glucose will be elevated as not all the insulin has been absorbed by the subcutaneous tissue. Topical insulin does not work! If insulin is seen on the surface of the skin, do not try to guesstimate what was lost and then re-inject more insulin. A safer plan would be to increase the frequency of monitoring and respond to elevated blood glucoses with corrective rapid-acting insulin every 2-3 hours until the blood glucose is restored to target.

If insulin consistently leaks from a site in spite of rotating injection sites carefully, here is a tip that often produces a positive outcome: after injecting, but prior to counting slowly to 5-10 and removing the needle, turn the needle a quarter twist before withdrawing.

Seeing blood at the injection site can be very scary for a child and worrisome for the parent. It is normal for you to feel that you have done something wrong or given a bad injection after seeing blood. Blood makes parents think that they have injected into a blood vessel or that blood mixed with insulin on the surface of the skin will lead to elevated blood glucose. If you have injected into the identified sites (as listed in Chapter 4: Insulin) rest assured that there are no major blood vessels that lie that close to the surface. It is important not to attempt to replace what appears to be lost insulin, but rather to increase frequency of monitoring and correct as needed for elevated blood glucoses.

Food

Food, glorious food, as Oliver Twist said, should be a source of pleasure and nourishment, as well as social interaction. In Chapter 7: Healthy Eating and Nutrition, you learned about healthy eating, the role of carbohydrates as an energy source and the importance of vitamins and minerals. For those with diabetes, food can also be a source of hyperglycemia if carbohydrate consumption does not match insulin, physical activity, or stress.

Today, it is more difficult than ever to estimate a portion size by looking at it on a dish or plate. Dish sizes have changed as well as what is considered the average portion size. It is a good idea to periodically take out scales and measuring cups/spoons to review the accuracy of the calculated carbohydrates. Miscalculated portions or carbohydrates can lead to underestimating the amount of rapid-acting insulin needed to cover a meal or snack and will lead to higher blood glucose readings. It is imperative to have a comprehensive carbohydrate reference book to use when there is no label on the package for review. The book should also include a breakdown of your child's favorite foods at their favorite fast food restaurant as well.

Carbohydrates that include a high fat content take longer to be broken down and digested. As a result, high-fat meals lead to high blood glucose readings even when the carbohydrate is accurately counted. The high fat meal may take as long as 4-6 hours to be broken down and digested. Rapid-acting insulin may last only 3-4 hours. Since there is no longer any insulin left to continue to lower the blood glucose level, it can lead to an elevated blood glucose reading.

In an effort to more accurately cover the carbohydrate content of a meal or snack, it may seem like a reasonable approach to consider giving rapid-acting insulin after eating, rather than before, to determine exactly what was eaten. It has been shown that this approach is *not* wise (except under specific circumstances, as discussed with your healthcare team) for several reasons.

- The carbohydrates within a meal will begin to raise the blood glucose within 15 minutes. As it takes rapid-acting insulin 15-30 minutes to be absorbed, the result is a mismatch of insulin effect to carbohydrate intake. It is recommended that insulin be administered 15-30 minutes prior to the meal to allow for the most effective coverage of carbohydrates.
- Planning to inject after a meal, rather than before, has the added risk of the insulin being missed altogether as a result of being distracted by getting on with the activities of the day.

Activity Levels

Seasonal differences in temperature and number of daylight hours, school year versus summer vacation, and age and developmental stage all affect activity levels. Does your child play a never ending game of baseball in the summer or do school and after school sports keep him or her more active during the school year? Do you live in an area with extreme temperatures (high and low) that make outdoor sports difficult at best, impossible at worst? Have computer games, social networking, and cell phones become the favored activities? As you read in Chapter 8: Physical Activity and Diabetes Management, exercise generates greater insulin sensitivity. With less activity, increases in insulin become necessary to prevent elevated blood glucoses.

It is necessary to have adequate insulin available for exercising muscles to access glucose. A blood glucose level should be checked prior to exercise. If the blood glucose level is greater than 250 mg/dL, it is important to check for ketones. If ketones are positive with an elevated blood glucose level, you need to correct the ketone and glucose levels before exercising. In the absence of adequate insulin, exercise will raise blood glucose levels. Therefore, it is helpful to talk with your diabetes healthcare team and read Chapter 8 prior to starting an exercise program.

Hormones

Just as your child outgrows shoes, she will outgrow her insulin dose. It is both normal and expected; you want your child to require more insulin, as it correlates to positive growth. The amount of change required will be variable, dependent on how rapid the growth is as well as the chronological age of the child. The rapid growth spurts of puberty will challenge your sense of how frequently and how aggressively doses need to be altered. The goal is to attempt to achieve blood glucose levels as close to near normal as possible. Growth hormone is only one of the hormones that impacts insulin sensitivity. It has been well studied that in the child *without* diabetes, the pancreas releases larger amounts of insulin when hormone levels increase. Other hormones that can affect the blood glucose are:

- Epinephrine: released as a result of severe emotional stress or physical pain
- Estrogen: changes before and during menses
- Dawn Phenomenon: the result of fading insulin levels and increased hormone levels (growth, epinephrine, glucagon) early in the morning
- Steroids: released as a result of illness and infection
- Adrenalin: released during exercise

Illness and Infection

When your child is sick or has an infection, it is not unusual for the blood glucose to rise. Do not forget to *check for ketones* if you suspect illness or infection. It is important for you to be alert to the following symptoms of infection or illness:

- Fever
- Pain or discomfort that a child can identify

- Nasal or sputum discharge that is green rather than clear
- Red, hot, swollen area or pus drainage from a wound/cut or insulin pump infusion site
- Vomiting

If your child has any of these symptoms, his or her blood glucose and ketone levels should be monitored as outlined in Chapter 11: Sick Days and DKA Prevention.

Medication

During illness and infection, there may be times when it is necessary to take medication. Some medications, such as adrenalin, cortisone, and prednisone will raise blood glucose. Check with your healthcare team if you have questions about over the counter medications and their effect on your child's blood glucose.

Hypoglycemia Resulting in Hyperglycemia?

Low blood glucose levels causing high blood levels? How is this possible? If a low blood glucose level (less than 70 mg/dL) is overtreated, the effect will then be elevated blood glucose. The Rule of 15 is that 15 grams of carb in 15 minutes will raise the blood glucose approximately 50 mg/dL. Given that the symptoms of low blood glucose often are hunger and a feeling of panic, it is easy to see how 4 ounces of juice can become juice, cookies, and anything else the refrigerator or cabinets have to offer. It is easy to overtreat — waiting 15 minutes for the carbohydrate to break down and raise the blood glucose can feel like the longest 15 minutes in history. Overtreating results in hyperglycemia an hour or so after the hypoglycemic episode. Your child ends up with yo-yo blood glucose levels.

In addition to over consumption of food, the blood glucose can rise if it falls below 70 mg/dL due to a counter-regulatory effect produced by the body. The body releases glucagon and epinephrine in response to the low blood glucose. Remember the above list of hormones that can raise the blood glucose? This effect of a high blood glucose level following a low blood glucose is referred to as the rebound (or Smogyi) effect.

Insulin Pumps

Causes for elevated blood glucoses as a result of a pump malfunction or user error is discussed extensively in Chapter 6: Insulin Pumps.

Insulin Dose Adjustments

Insulin doses change and require adjustments for a variety of reasons. The ability to make adjustments to insulin doses gives you and your child better outcomes in terms of diabetes management. With time, experience, and help from your diabetes healthcare team, you should be able to make dose adjustments to prevent hyperglycemia. Generally, doses are adjusted by 10% increments. Insulin adjustments are typically made during your child's honeymoon phase, periods of growth, puberty, change in physical activity, illness, and times such as holiday gatherings. When making an insulin adjustment, consider the following:

1. Look for patterns that appear over 3-5 days. For example, perhaps dinner or breakfast readings are continuously elevated.
2. Consider what type of insulin your child is on, its onset, peak, and duration. For instance, rapid-acting insulin is what affects blood glucose after a meal.
3. Adjust insulin dose in a 10% increment
4. Rule out other causes of hyperglycemia (*i.e*,. illness, hypoglycemic rebound, etc.)
5. Adjust one insulin type at a time
6. Record dose adjustments in your logbook
7. Take time to practice dose adjustments with your diabetes health-care team.

When to Seek Help

Even with excellent diabetes education, there are times when you must seek help from your healthcare team. Diabetes education should provide you with the ability to manage hyperglycemia situations, but there are times when additional guidance is needed. The following are examples of times when you should call your diabetes healthcare team:

- Continuous blood glucose above target range, despite multiple insulin dose changes
- The presence of urine ketones that are small, medium, or large, or blood ketones that are greater than 0.6mmol/L. Ketone testing should be done when blood glucose readings are greater than 250 mg/dL for 2 tests in a row, or during illness
- Fever, illness, or infection
- When there is a suspicion of diabetic ketoacidosis (DKA).
  - The signs and symptoms of DKA include:
    - Dehydration
    - Extreme thirst
    - Nausea
    - Decreased appetite
    - Rapid weight loss
    - Vomiting
    - Stomach pain
    - Chest pain
    - Fruity odor to the breath (acetone)
    - Rapid shallow breathing (Kussmaul respirations)
    - Sleepiness

Summary

Though the goal is to have blood glucose levels in your child's target range as much as possible, hyperglycemia will occur. Remember that long-term complications do not occur due to a high blood glucose level here or there. Knowing the reasons why hyperglycemia occurs provides you with tools to decrease the highs. Developing problem solving techniques, based on previous experience, will help you adjust blood glucose levels into your child's target range with greater accuracy and frequency.

References and Resources

Lawlor M, Laffel L, Anderson B, Bertorelli A. *Caring for Young Children Living with Diabetes: Professional Manual.* Boston, MA: Joslin Diabetes Center, 1996.

Laffel L, Pasquarello C, Lawlor M. Treatment of the child and adolescent with diabetes. In: Kahn CR, Weir GC, King GL, Jacobson AM, Moses AC, Smith RJ, editors. *Joslin's Diabetes Mellitus*. Philadelphia: Lippincott Williams & Wilkins, 2005: 711-736.

Laffel L. Sick-day management in type 1 diabetes. *Endocrinol Metab Clin North Am*. 2000; 29(4):707-723.

Web sites:

- www.diabetes.org
- Joslin Diabetes Center: www.joslin.org
- American Diabetes Association: www.diabetes.org
- Children with Diabetes: www.childrenwithdiabetes.com

11

Sick Days and DKA Prevention

As a parent, you know that illness, infection, emotional stress, and physical stresses, such as surgery or injury, are all part of childhood and adolescence. For youth with type 1 diabetes, these events can lead to poor metabolic control. Poor control can also be caused by events related to diabetes, such as insulin pump failure, a missed insulin dose, or spoiled insulin. The results can include: elevated blood glucose levels, ketonuria (ketones in the urine), dehydration, and diabetic ketoacidosis (DKA). Alternatively, with vomiting and diarrhea resulting from illness (*e.g.*, stomach flu, etc.), hypoglycemia may occur because of decreased eating and poor absorption of nutrients. Thus, sick-day management requires increased monitoring of blood glucose, urine, or blood monitoring for ketones, as well as attention to other diabetes management tasks.

This chapter will provide guidelines on how to handle diabetes management in the event your child is ill or injured. We will focus on maintaining good metabolic control through the use of sick-day guidelines and protocols. We will also review the importance of sick-day management and provide information to help you keep your child well. Remember — your diabetes healthcare team is a necessary resource when your child is ill and experiencing high blood glucose levels and ketones. They are always just a call away.

Sick-Day Guidelines

An illness can increase levels of the counter-regulatory hormones glucagon, adrenaline, growth hormone, and cortisol. The result is hyperglycemia (high blood glucose) due to both insulin resistance and increased production and release of glucose by the liver. When your child has hyperglycemia, he doesn't have enough insulin to use the glucose in his body. Given this, he must first be treated with insulin. When your child is suffering from an infection, such as bronchitis, strep throat, or urinary tract infection, this release of hormones may interfere with normal insulin action or produce resistance to the insulin. Similarly, stress can increase hormones that increase blood glucose levels and cause resistance to insulin. Clearly, if insulin is not given, or is missed due to an insulin pump problem such as blocked tubing, or if the insulin has spoiled due to overheating or freezing, there will not be enough insulin in the body. (If you suspect insulin is spoiled, open a new bottle or cartridge.) With the help of your diabetes healthcare team, you will be better able to take care of your child when sick days occur. To get started, let's learn the sick-day rules.

Sick-Day Rules

Sick-day rules provide steps to treat high blood glucose levels and ketones resulting from illness or injury. The *goals* of sick-day rules are to:

- Treat high blood glucose levels
- Reduce or prevent ketones
- Prevent diabetic ketoacidosis (DKA)
- Prevent or treat low blood glucose levels

Table 11-1 lists sick-day rules to follow if your child is ill.

Table 11-1. Sick-Day Rules
• Always give insulin — the dose may need to be changed with the help of your diabetes healthcare team
• Drink fluids to prevent dehydration
• Continue eating or adjust insulin doses to prevent hypoglycemia
• Monitor blood glucose
• Monitor blood or urine ketones
• Give additional fast-acting or rapid-acting insulin based on your diabetes healthcare team guidelines
• Treat the underlying illness/injury
• Call your diabetes healthcare team for support and guidance

What makes sick days different?

Sick days make themselves known either by hyperglycemia (high blood glucose) on blood glucose checks or by symptoms of hyperglycemia (thirst, increased urination, blurred vision, mood swings, hunger, weight loss or poor weight gain, and/or nausea and/or vomiting.) Prolonged hyperglycemia can result in fluid loss and dehydration. Fever, vomiting, and diarrhea further increase the loss of fluids and the risk of dehydration. Your child may complain of stomach pain or seem lethargic. There may be signs of infection such as fever, headache, rash, sore throat, cough, or painful urination.

As the illness or lack of insulin continues, *ketones* begin to appear in the blood and in the urine. If your child's body does not have enough insulin to use its glucose, or if other hormones such as adrenaline, cortisol, or growth hormone are high, his or her body will produce ketones. There are three ketones: Beta-hydroxybutyrate (BOH), acetoacetate, and acetone. BOH, is measured in the blood using a blood ketone meter (similar to measuring blood glucose). BOH is measured in millimoles/L (mmol/L). A level greater than 0.5 mmol/L is considered high and indicates a need to take action. Levels below that can occur if you haven't eaten in awhile, such as first thing in the morning. Urine ketones measure acetoacetate using a strip which is dipped in urine. Many urine strips measure ketones based on a scale of negative, trace, small, moderate or large (1+ to 4+). Ketones appear in the blood before they can be measured in the urine. Ketones also disappear more quickly in the blood than in the urine after insulin treatment. In addition, ketones may continue to be present in the urine many hours after they have been cleared from the blood, potentially leading to the provision of unnecessary extra insulin. You may smell ketones on your child's breath, as the body tries to get rid of them through the lungs. The odor is usually described as sweet or fruity, and this odor represents the ketone acetone.

Diabetic Ketoacidosis (DKA)

Ketones are acids, thus diabetic ketoacidosis, or DKA, results when the amount of ketones in the blood rises beyond the point where the body is able to compensate for the extra acids. Ketones will persist until the insulin level is once again high enough to shut off their production. Symptoms of DKA include stomach upset, vomiting, difficult or rapid breathing, and changes in alertness. A person with DKA has significant chemical imbalances that may require hospitalization or become life-threatening.

Who is at risk for DKA?

Any individual who has type 1 diabetes, and even some with type 2 diabetes, are at risk for DKA. If your child's ketone level is very high, usually his or her blood glucose level will also be high. The risk is greatest when diabetes, although present, has not yet been diagnosed. With established diabetes, the risk for DKA is greater when insulin is missed and blood glucose and ketone checks are infrequent (especially if using an insulin pump and a dislodged catheter goes unrecognized). In these cases, the occurrence of an infection or other stress may tip the balance toward DKA. Early recognition of high ketone and blood glucose levels and the correct responses are keys to the prevention of DKA. One of the primary responses should be to call your diabetes healthcare team. You should never be afraid to call for help and direction from your diabetes healthcare team; they are here to help you and want to be called.

What about illnesses with vomiting and diarrhea?

Illnesses where vomiting and diarrhea are the primary signs may present with unusually low blood glucoses (sometimes starting just before the actual illness) and ketones. The hypoglycemia and the ketones are the result of the body's inability to absorb nutrition, so in this case, the insulin dose may actually have to be decreased (but not eliminated). Dehydration from vomiting, diarrhea, fever and lack of intake is a common problem.

Management of Sick Days

Is it a Sick Day? Assess the Blood Glucose and Ketone Levels

If your child's blood glucose is over 250 mg/dL and ketones are positive (blood ketones: 0.6 mmol/L or higher or urine ketones: more than a trace), it is a sick day and a cause and treatment should be determined. *Remember* — your diabetes healthcare team is there to help and should be contacted.

If the level of blood ketones is 0.6-0.9 mmol/L or the level of urine

Table 11-2. Determine the Cause for Hyperglycemia and Ketones

Determine a cause: When blood glucose is greater than 250 mg/dL and ketones are present
• Is there an infection? Fever, flu-symptoms, vomiting, or diarrhea? • Did you or your child forget or omit an insulin dose? Take a smaller dose than usual? • Is your child under a lot of stress? • Was a meal or snack missed? • Did the insulin go bad? Exposure to temperatures less than 40°F or greater than 86°F
If your child is on an insulin pump:
• Did the cannula come out of the skin? • Is there air in the tubing? • Is the pump suspended? • Is the pump attached and working? • Is there insulin in the pump?

Table 11-3. Determine a Treatment for Hyperglycemia and Ketones

Determine a treatment: When blood glucose is greater than 250 mg/dL and ketones are present
• *Remember—always give insulin!*
• Supplemental insulin dose: since your child will often need more insulin than normal when ill, injured, or stressed, an extra or supplemental dose or doses of insulin is often necessary.
• Rapid-acting insulin (lispro, aspart, glulisine) is the insulin used for extra doses of insulin.
• Insulin injections or pump boluses can be repeated every 2-3 hours to clear ketones and to maintain blood glucose levels at approximately 100–200 mg/dL. Intermediate- and long-acting insulins (NPH, glargine, detemir) should be given as usual. – Calculate your child's Total Daily Dose (TDD): Refer to Tables 11-4 (urine ketones) or 11-5 (blood ketones) to decide if your child needs supplemental insulin. If so, calculate your child's average TDD: • *If on injections:* Add up the total number of units of insulin your child takes each day. To figure out the number of units to use for a sliding scale bolus dose, use the average or lower number. For example, if at lunch the dose is 4–6 units, use 5 for the number to be added. If the dose is 4-7 units, use 5 units for the number to be added. • *If on insulin pump:* Look at the memory to see if the TDD is normally about the same; if so, use a rounded off number. If the TDD is not similar from day to day, ask your diabetes healthcare team to calculate a TDD by using your basal/bolus regimen, correction factor, sensitivity factor and target glucose level. – Calculate the supplemental insulin dose: Use Table 11-4 or 11-5 to find the percentage you need to calculate the supplemental dose. Multiply the TDD by that percentage to determine the supplemental dose of rapid-acting insulin. *Example:* TDD = 20; Blood glucose = 352 mg/dL; Blood ketone = 1.2 mmol/L; % extra = 10%; Supplemental Dose = TDD x % from table = 20 x 10% = 2 units of rapid acting insulin

Table 11-4. Supplemental Insulin Dosages Using Urine Ketone Results

Supplemental Rapid-Acting Insulin Dosages Using Urine Ketone Results			
Urine Ketones	Blood Glucose Level (mg/dL)*		
	Less than 250	250-400	Greater than 400
Negative or Trace	No extra	10%	10–15%
Small, Medium or Large	0%	15%	20%

Table 11-5. Supplemental Insulin Dosages Using Blood Ketone Results

Supplemental Rapid-Acting Insulin Dosages Using Blood Ketone Results			
Blood Ketones (mmol/L)	Blood Glucose Level (mg/dL)		
	Less than 250	250-400	Greater than 400
Less than 1.0	No change	5%	10%
1.0–1.4	0% to 5%	10%	15%
Greater than 1.5	0% to 10%	15% to 20%	20%

ketones is small, recheck for ketones in 2 to 4 hours after starting treatment; if the blood level is greater than or equal to 3.0 mmol/L or the urine level is greater than medium, call your healthcare team immediately.

If the blood glucose level is less than 80 mg/dL and your child cannot eat or keep food down, leave out rapid-acting acting insulin and decrease intermediate-/long-acting insulin by 20%. Contact your healthcare team, especially if vomiting or if blood glucose levels remain under 80 mg/dL.

If your child has ketones and is also experiencing a poor appetite, vomiting, or diarrhea and the blood glucose is normal to low, the ketones are likely to be starvation ketones and are often accompanied with dehydration. You will need to provide fluids, calories, and insulin, unless the blood glucose is falling or low. Glucose-containing fluids (see list under *Sick-Day Cabinet* later in this chapter) are usually the best way to go, using small but frequent amounts. The amounts suggested in the Table 11-6 will help to keep your child hydrated, and help the body to stop

Table 11-6. Minimal Replacement Fluids Based on Weight

Weight in Pounds	Ounces per Hour
Less than 40	2 oz
40–120	3 oz
Greater than 120	4 oz

producing starvation ketones. If your child cannot take fluids, he or she may need to receive them intravenously, and this will often cause a rapid improvement.

Prevent Dehydration

Fluids prevent dehydration and assist the body in clearing ketones. Preventing dehydration will keep your child more comfortable and less prone to increasing ketones. Liquids should be sugar-free if blood glucose is greater than 200 mg/dL, but may contain sugar if blood glucose is less than 200 mg/dL and your child is not eating. Liquids such as Pedialyte, broth, or soup help restore salt and other electrolytes that have been lost by vomiting or excess urination. In a child with an upset stomach, fluids should be given in small quantities (sips) to discourage vomiting. Table 11-6 shows recommended *minimal* amounts of fluids give to your child based on the child's size. These are guidelines only. If such additional fluids are necessary, call your healthcare team. The team will make an assessment and let you know how and when to provide your child with fluids. If your child is unable to take in this minimal amount, IV fluids may be recommended. See *Sick-Day Cabinet* later in this chapter for suggestions of fluids to have on hand.

Frequent Monitoring

Blood glucose should be checked every 2-3 hours, sometimes as often as every hour initially. Ketones should also be checked every 2-3 hours until

Table 11-7. Sick-Day Questions to Answer and Track:

Please record the following information every 2 hours:							
Please record a "Start Time":	Start	Hr2	Hr4	Hr6	Hr8	Hr10	Hr12
Blood glucose							
Ketones (check one) ☐ BLOOD ☐ URINE							
Insulin dose							
Weight							
Food							
Fluids (in ounces)							
Call your healthcare team if symptoms persist more than 6-12 hours or if your child vomits more then once.							

they are negative. You should see a steady decrease in both blood glucose and ketones. It is helpful to keep a written record (see Table 11-7) of blood glucoses, ketones, and fluids. This record will help you when you talk with your diabetes healthcare team.

Treat the Underlying Illness

Any other illness must be treated. Medications (either over-the-counter or prescription), rest, fluids, etc., may all be part of the treatment plan. For most children, diabetes does not alter the usual treatments for other illnesses. In general, antibiotic drugs and over-the-counter medications may contain very little sugar and can be used by children with diabetes. If your child has a high blood glucose level while on medication, the elevated glucose is probably due to the underlying illness and not the medication. One exception is the use of steroids (like prednisone) which may be given to your child for severe asthma or poison ivy. Steroids cause your child to need extra larger-than-normal doses of insulin. Steroids should be used with great caution and only with a doctor's prescription and supervision. Most medications will be prescribed by your regular primary care physician; if you have any questions concerning a medication's effect on diabetes management, remember to ask your primary care provider or your diabetes healthcare team.

Contact Your Diabetes Healthcare Team

When your child was diagnosed with diabetes, part of the education provided was sick-day management; ongoing education reviewed the topic. However, you may not have encountered a sick day before, or you may need to discuss how to manage this particular event. Contact your healthcare team when:

- Your child is ill and you need to review Sick-Day Rules
- Blood glucose is elevated and/or ketones are present
- There is persistent illness for over 4-6 hours; frequent diarrhea; vomiting more than once; refusing fluids
- Your child has signs of dehydration — dry lips and mouth, sunken eyes, dry skin, and weight loss

- Signs or symptoms of infection
- Change in appearance, alertness, breathing, pain
- You need advice on how much insulin to give
- Hypoglycemia resulting from illness or treatment

Vomiting, Diarrhea and Hypoglycemia

Loss of fluids and electrolytes from vomiting and diarrhea, and poor intake of nutrients can result in ketones as well as low blood glucose. Calories, especially from carbohydrates, are necessary along with insulin to stop further increases in ketones, to treat low blood glucose and dehydration. In this case, whether given by mouth at home or by IV at a medical facility, fluids should contain sugar. Please refer to Chapter 9: Hypoglycemia, where we covered the topics of *Glucagon* and *Mini-Dose Glucagon*. Glucagon is a medical treatment for severe hypoglycemia (low blood glucose). Severe hypoglycemia can occur due to illness, injury, or stress and thus glucagon may be needed. Because insulin doses may have to be changed, it is wise to be in touch with your healthcare team.

Sick-Day Nutrition Guidelines

Sick days are a challenging time for parents and children. Below are some nutrition guidelines to help you through your child's illness.

- **Fluids:** Your child should drink 6-8 oz of fluid every 1 to 2 hours to prevent dehydration (too much fluid loss as a result of diarrhea, stomach upset or high temperature). Select what your child prefers to drink from the following list:
  - Sugar free, caffeine free-soda* (e.g., diet ginger ale, diet Sprite, diet 7-Up)
  - Crystal Light or sugar-free Kool Aid
  - Decaffeinated tea (Caffeine causes the loss of fluids more rapidly through urination and should be avoided)
  - Water (Fruit 2 O, spring water, seltzer water)
  - Sugar-free Jell-O

- Clear liquids, such as Jell-O, soda, broth, and apple juice may be easier to tolerate than creamier items when your child is feeling sick to his or her stomach.

Foods for Replacing Carbohydrate

If your child is unable to follow his or her meal plan when sick, you should replace at least the carbohydrate portions of the meal plan. Provide 1-2 of these items (see Table 11-8) every 1-2 hours (each item is equal to approximately 10-15 grams of carbohydrate per serving). Always check the carbohydrate content on the food label.

Pediatric Rehydration Solutions are also available at supermarkets and drug stores. They can be used when your child is having difficulty keeping anything down. They contain some carbohydrate so please read the label carefully. Listed below are a few examples.

- **Enfalyte** (Mead Johnson) 8 oz = 30 calories, 7.5 grams carbohydrate
- **Pedialyte** (Ross) 8 oz = 24 calories, 6 grams carbohydrate
- **Pedialyte Freezer Pops** (Ross) 1 each (2.1 fluid ounces) = 6 calories, 1.5 grams carbohydrate

Table 11-8. Foods for Replacing Carbohydrate

Applesauce	½ c	Hot cereal	½ c
Apple juice	½ c	Italian Ice	½ c
Baby cereal (dry)	½ c	Lifesavers (large size)	3–4 each
Baby food fruit	3–4 oz	Lifesavers (regular size)	½ roll
Banana (small)	1 each	Crème Savers	3–4 each
Chocolate milk	½ c	Lollipop (Jolly Rancher)	1 each
Chocolate syrup	2 tsp	Milkshake	¼ c
Cranberry juice (white)	½ c	Orange juice	½ c
Eggnog	½ c	Regular Jell-O®	½ c
Gatorade	1 cup	Regular ice cream	½ c
Go-gurt	1 tube	Regular pudding	¼ c
Grape juice (white)	⅓ c	Sherbert	¼ c
Fruited yogurt	⅓ c	Twin pop popsicle	1 pop
Honey	1 Tbsp		

Other food choices that you may try include salty foods like broth, consommé, tomato juice, or soft solids like toast, hot cereals or soups.

If your child is unable to take liquids because of a stomach ache, he or she is throwing up, is in pain, or if you are unsure of what to do, *call your healthcare team for help*.

The Sick-Day Cabinet

Having supplies ready in case of emergency will allow you to treat your child more confidently and earlier. Caretakers should know where supplies are kept and the contents should be reviewed from time to time to ensure they are up to date and complete. Items suggested for your sick-day cabinet include:

- A copy of the sick-day rules
- Blood glucose meter and strips
- Ketone strips (urine and/or blood)
- Glucagon kit
- Thermometer
- Aspirin-free products in liquid, chewable and/or suppository form
- Regular and sugar free soda
- Broth or bullion
- Regular and sugar-free drinks, such as juice boxes, and drink bags/boxes. Popular brands and types include Kool-Aid, Capri Sun, HiC, electrolyte sport drinks (Gatorade, Propel, G2, Powerade) etc.
- Regular and sugar-free Jell-O
- Commercially available rehydration fluids designed for the age of your child
- Emergency telephone numbers

Surgery

In the event that your child has a scheduled surgical procedure, speak with your child's pediatric endocrinologist as soon as you schedule the surgery. Your child's healthcare team will individualize any guidelines necessary. General guidelines for surgery are available from your diabetes healthcare team.

Summary

Illness, injury, stress, surgery, pump failure, and spoiled insulin are all factors that can lead to a "sick day." As blood glucose levels rise and ketones accumulate it is very important to take action immediately. Use this chapter as a guide to avert serious deteriorization in diabetes management. Do not hesitate to contact your diabetes healthcare team for medical advice.

References and Resources

Brink S, et al. Sick day management in children and adolescents with diabetes. *Pediatric Diabetes*. 2007:8:401-407.

Laffel, L Sick-day management in type 1 diabetes. *Endocrinology and Metabolism Clinics of North America*. 2000:29(4):707-723.

Bismuth E, Svoren B, Volkening L, Butler D, Laffel L. Impact of insulin pump therapy and blood b-OHB ketone monitoring on glycemic outcomes in youth with type 1 diabetes (T1D) [Abstract]. *Diabetes*. 2007; 56 (Suppl 1):A485.

Wolfsdorf J, Glaser N, Sperling MA. Diabetic ketoacidosis in infants, children, and adolescents: A consensus statement from the American Diabetes Association. *Diabetes Care*. 2006; 29(5):1150-1159.

Web sites:

- Joslin Diabetes Center: www.joslin.org
- American Diabetes Association: www.diabetes.org
- Juvenile Diabetes Research Foundation: www.jdrf.org
- Children With Diabetes: www.childrenwithdiabetes.com

12

Physical Growth and Development in Adolescents with Diabetes

Physical growth and sexual development affect diabetes management in children and teens. This chapter focuses on the effect of growth and hormones on insulin requirements, bone health, and reproductive health issues for teens.

Growth during Childhood and Puberty

Children grow very rapidly in their first year of life. Growth, both in terms of weight and length/height, slows down over the next two years, and from ages 3 to 9, children grow about 2 inches in height each year. Figure 12-1 shows an example of a Growth Chart from the Center for Disease Control and Prevention. Additional growth charts can be found at: www.brightfutures.org/bf2/pdf/pdf/GrowthCharts.pdf

Your child's height and weight is plotted on a growth chart to record ongoing growth. You and your child's pediatric team as well as his or her diabetes healthcare team watch for any deviations from the normal. This way, all are aware of any potential problems which may have to be addressed.

Physical Changes and Growth during Puberty

Growth rate increases as teens enter their pubertal growth spurt. Some guidelines for puberty are shown in Table 12-1.

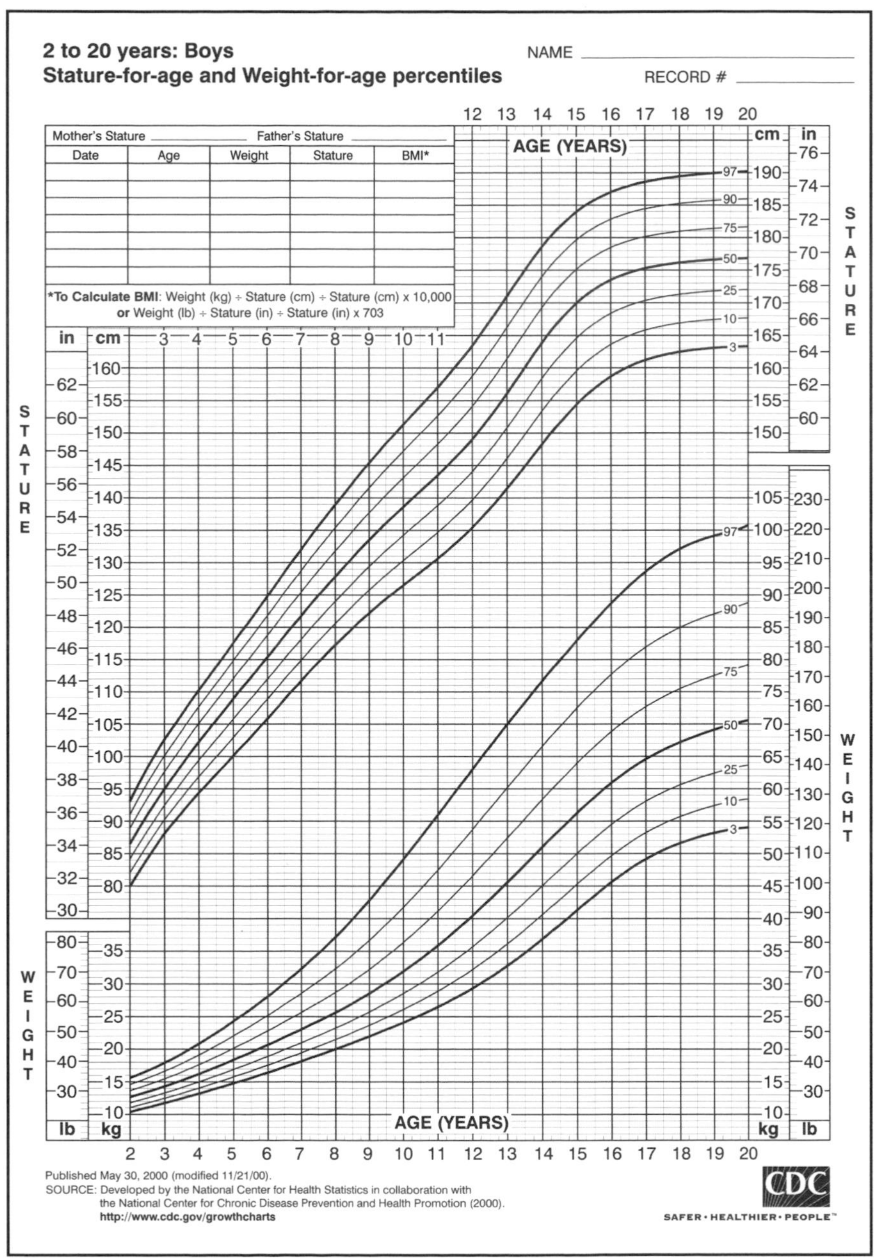

Figure 12-1. Sample Growth Chart

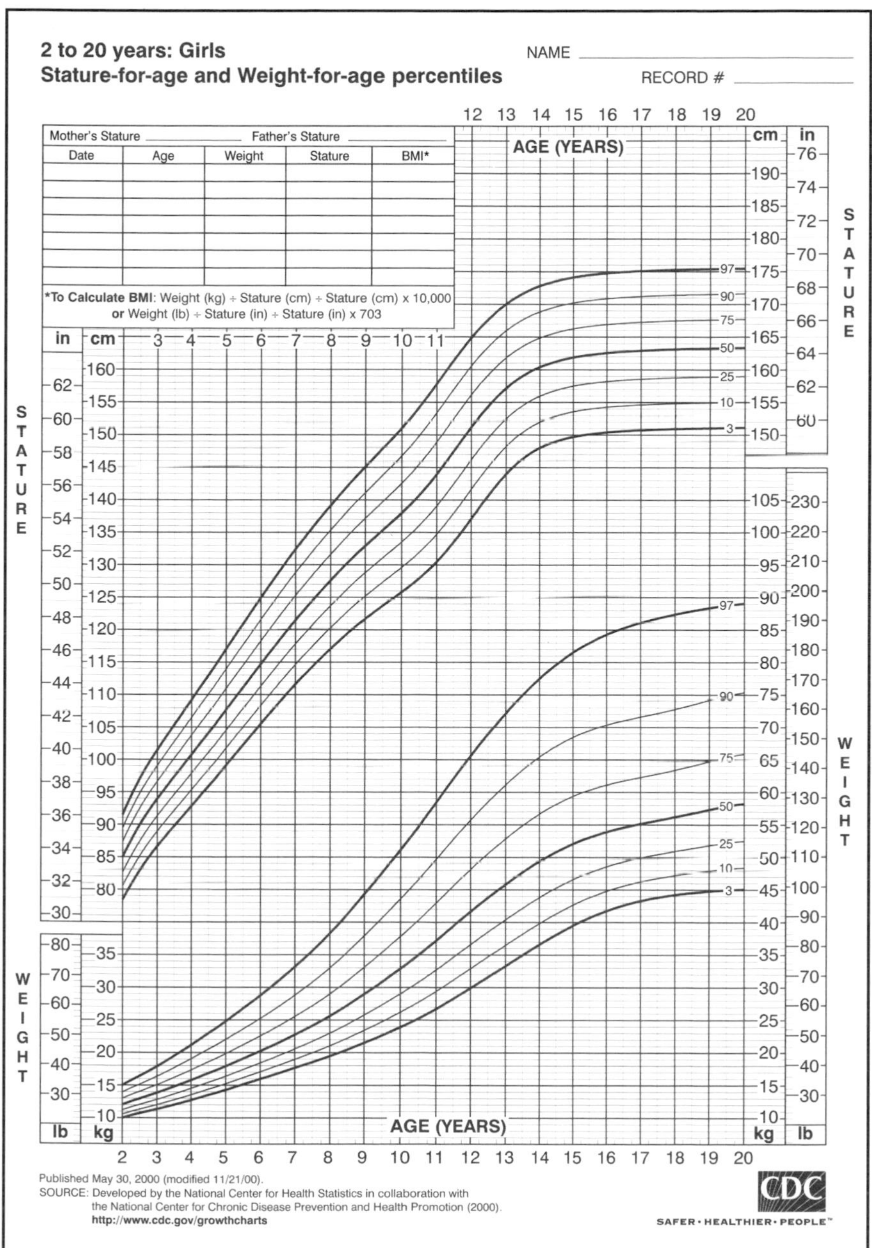
2 to 20 years: Girls
Stature-for-age and Weight-for-age percentiles
NAME
RECORD #
Mother's Stature
Father's Stature
Date
Age
Weight
Stature
BMI*
*To Calculate BMI: Weight (kg) ÷ Stature (cm) ÷ Stature (cm) x 10,000
or Weight (lb) ÷ Stature (in) ÷ Stature (in) x 703
AGE (YEARS)
STATURE
WEIGHT
97
90
75
50
25
10
3
cm
in
kg
lb
Published May 30, 2000 (modified 11/21/00).
SOURCE: Developed by the National Center for Health Statistics in collaboration with the National Center for Chronic Disease Prevention and Health Promotion (2000).
http://www.cdc.gov/growthcharts
CDC
SAFER · HEALTHIER · PEOPLE™

Table 12-1. Guidelines for Growth during Puberty

Girls	Boys
Puberty begins for girls with breast development at an average age of just under 10 years in Caucasian girls in the United States.	Puberty begins for boys with testicular enlargement at an average age of 11 years but it is normal for this to happen between the ages of 9 to 14.
Girls enter puberty about two years earlier than boys, so that in junior high school, girls are often taller and stronger than the boys in their class.	If your son has not had any pubertal development by age 14, he should be evaluated by his healthcare provider.
Girls reach their greatest height velocity of about 3½ inches per year at an average age of 12 years.	Boys reach their greatest height velocity of about 4 inches per year at an average age of 14 years (3 years after puberty begins).
Girls growth rate begins to speed up as breast development begins. • They continue to grow in height until they are about 15 years old on average, adding about 2 inches in height after periods have started. • Menstrual cycles (periods) start at an average age of 12½ years. — The normal range for starting periods is between the ages of 10-15 years. • African American and Latino girls: — Start breast development about 6 months earlier than Caucasian girls. — Breast development or pubic hair development under age 8 is more common in African American girls.	Boys reach their peak strength spurt with: • Broadening of their shoulders. • Increased muscle development around the age of 15 (late in the overall process of male puberty). • Gradual increase of testosterone and estrogen as male puberty proceeds. • Appearance of pubic and underarm hair and enlargement of the penis. • Deepening of the voice and the start of nocturnal emissions. • Development of small breast buds for many boys during mid puberty which go away as the growth spurt slows.
Early puberty is more common in girls. • Girls who have breast development or pubic hair under age 8 years are generally considered to have early puberty. Usually this is a normal variant, although some serious medical conditions can present as early puberty.	Early puberty is less common in boys.
Delayed puberty is less common in girls. • Girls who have no breast development by age 13 should be evaluated.	Delayed puberty is more common in boys. • Often the pattern of late puberty runs in a family.

Muscle, Fat, and Bone Growth

The relative amount of muscle, fat, and bone in a child's body changes as the child grows. Infants and toddlers have a greater percentage of their weight as body fat than older children. In girls, body fat decreases from age 3-6 years and begins to increase after age 6, continuing to increase throughout life. Girls carry an average of 10 more pounds of body fat at the same height at age 18 years than at 13 years. On average, women carry twice the percentage of body fat as men, which give women the energy stores needed to support pregnancy and breast feeding an infant. Girls need about 2,500 calories a day during their peak growth spurt, but as growth slows after the age of 13, baseline energy needs decrease to an average of 1,500 calories a day.

Weight Concerns in Girls with Diabetes

It is very helpful for girls with diabetes whose growth is slowing down, to continue to see a nutritionist yearly after their growth spurt, to receive guidance in decreasing their caloric intake as they transition to healthy adult eating habits. Some girls with diabetes become overweight for their height if they do not decrease their food intake and their insulin doses after their growth in height begins to slow. This is a difficult time for girls, as they are often very concerned and dissatisfied with their body at this stage of adolescence. (See Chapter 13: Diabetes and Family Issues, for additional information on disordered eating/eating disorders.) The images that adolescents see of models in teen magazines, on television, and in the movies show emaciated women as role models for physical attractiveness. As a result, some teen girls become excessively concerned about their body weight. This can evolve into a disordered eating/eating disorder in some girls. Girls with diabetes are at special risk for disordered eating/eating disorders. The issue of weight needs to be addressed cautiously and with support. It is easy for a parent or healthcare team member to inadvertently contribute to the development of an eating disorder by excessively focusing on weight issues in a young woman in this early adolescent stage of development.

Girls with diabetes sometimes skip an insulin dose or take less insulin than prescribed to keep their weight low. This can result in very poor diabetes control. These girls need counseling to help them develop a more positive body image. The pattern of insulin underdosing and omission can become a lifelong habit with very negative effects on long-term diabetes control. Girls and women who chronically underdose insulin to control weight are at high risk for complications of diabetes and are endangering their lives. It is very important for parents and the diabetes healthcare team to help the young woman who is skimping on insulin for weight control. The behavior must be addressed as a very serious health threatening issue and adults need to problem solve with her to identify ways to take a more positive approach to feeling in control of her body.

Increase in Insulin Requirements during Puberty

Insulin requirements increase dramatically as children enter their pubertal growth spurt. The hormones of puberty — estrogen and testosterone — increase insulin resistance so that more insulin is needed to keep blood glucose in range. Growth hormone also increases during puberty and causes insulin resistance. Since growth hormone is made primarily during sleep, insulin resistance and insulin needs increase during the early morning hours, from about 3 am to 10 am. Growing children make different amounts of growth hormone on different nights, so insulin needs vary from night to night during puberty, causing more variable morning blood glucose in teens. The breakfast rapid-acting insulin dose may need to be larger than the insulin doses needed for meals later in the day due to the early morning insulin resistance. Teens in their growth spurt typically need one-and-a-half times the insulin dose per pound of body weight as compared to younger children. Parents are often surprised by how much teens eat during their growth spurt. Girls need an average of 2,500 calories a day during their growth spurt, and boys need 4,000 calories. The timing of insulin onsets, peaks, and durations needs to match the timing of the food intake. Using meal time insulin doses based on insulin-to-carbohydrate ratios can help teens to satisfy their hunger during their growth spurt while maintaining optimal blood glucose control and maximizing the absorption of calories needed for growth. Children and teens whose blood glucose control is very poor due to not enough insulin (because they are taking too little insulin or frequently missing insulin doses), may grow poorly and have delayed or poorly progressing puberty. Their bodies think that they are starving since the food that is eaten cannot enter the cells of the body to be used as energy without enough insulin. If this happens, these children lose weight or fail to gain weight normally and grow poorly. Some studies have shown that teens with diabetes have a slightly later onset of puberty and onset of menstrual cycling than teens without diabetes, but if your child's diabetes is well controlled, puberty can be expected to progress normally unless there is another reason for delayed or interrupted puberty.

Medical Conditions that May Affect Growth

Medical conditions that result in poor absorption of food may also cause poor growth. If children have untreated celiac disease (sensitivity to gluten in foods) or untreated inflammatory bowel disease, they will often grow poorly and have delayed puberty. These children will have symptoms of pain, diarrhea, or gas after eating, and they may eat less to avoid discomfort after eating. Most often, teens with celiac disease lose weight or fail to gain weight normally, but some are overweight for their height. These teens may overeat, perhaps as attempt to relieve intestinal discomfort.

Sometimes teens who are worried that they are overweight cut back their food intake so much that they grow poorly. This is most common in girls who feel that they are fat even when they are losing too much weight and becoming too thin to grow. Disordered eating/eating disorders do occur in teens with diabetes and can seriously complicate diabetes management.

Growing Strong Bones

Bones increase in size and density during adolescence. In girls, this occurs early in puberty. Between ages 10-18 years, the amount of calcium in bones doubles in girls. Bone density and the amount of calcium in bone continues to increase in women until they reach their mid twenties, and gradually declines after that. Many young women do not get enough calcium and vitamin D during their growing years to give them maximum bone density. Although thin bones are more common in girls than boys, boys and men can also have thin bones. Growing girls and boys need 1,200 mg of calcium a day. This is equal to the amount of calcium in 5 servings of dairy products a day or, if they are unable or unwilling to get enough calcium in their meal plan, the same as taking 600 mg of a calcium supplement twice a day. In addition to calcium, vitamin D is needed to absorb calcium from the diet. Vitamin D is made in the skin in the summer; however, many people are low in vitamin D in the winter months. Children and teens should get 400-800 units of vitamin D a day. A multivitamin has 400 units of vitamin D, and a quart of milk has 400 units of vitamin D. Many calcium supplements also have added 200 units of vitamin D with 600 mg of calcium. You may want your child to take one of these chewable supplements twice a day to provide full calcium and vitamin D supplementation. There have been some studies suggesting that osteoporosis (thin bones due to low levels of calcium in bone) is more common in people with diabetes than in the general population, so that is why it is important to ensure that your child is receiving an adequate amount of calcium and vitamin D.

Hormones and Growth

Children need growth hormone and thyroid hormone to grow. During puberty children also require the hormones estrogen and testosterone for normal growth. Growth hormone deficiency is rare. Children who completely lack growth hormone or who do not respond to growth hormone grow extremely slowly, and typically grow less than 2 inches a year. Most often these children are below the growth chart from early childhood onwards. Growth hormone is usually made mostly during sleep, but the proteins that are made in response to growth hormone, like IgF1(insulin like growth factor 1) and IgFBP3 (insulin growth factor binding protein 3) can be measured in a blood test in the child who is suspected of having growth hormone deficiency. Stimulation testing of growth hormone can be done by an endocrinologist if necessary. Growth hormone can be replaced by daily injection in the rare situation that a child does not make growth hormone normally on his or her own.

Much more commonly, children with diabetes may grow poorly because they have low thyroid hormone levels and it is this hormone that supports normal metabolism throughout the body. This occurs in up to 10% of children with type 1 diabetes. In people who have a tendency toward autoimmune problems, the thyroid gland can by attacked by the immune system, which causes inflammation in the thyroid. This is called thyroiditis. Sometimes the thyroid gland in front of the neck becomes enlarged. This is called a goiter. Children with thyroiditis usually have thyroid antibodies which can be measured on a blood test. Thyroid function can also be easily measured with a blood test. In some people with thyroiditis, the thyroid will not secrete enough thyroid hormone.

If thyroid hormone is low, a person may have some or all of the following symptoms:

- Feel tired
- Feel cold easily

- Have dry skin
- Have increased hair loss when brushing their hair
- Have a slower heart rate
- Have lower blood pressure
- Be constipated
- Have a decreased appetite but may have increase in body weight
- Have slowed growth in height
- Have delayed puberty
- In girls, periods may stop or may become too frequent and heavy

Since thyroid problems due to thyroiditis are relatively common in children with diabetes, thyroid hormone screening is usually done once a year. If thyroid hormone is low, it is easily replaced with a thyroid supplement pill that can be taken once a day. Initially, the dose is adjusted with a blood test for thyroid function, then 4-6 weeks after starting the thyroid replacement, and every 6 months once the correct dose is determined.

The hormones estrogen, testosterone, and the adrenal androgen hormones are important in growth and puberty. In mid-childhood, around the ages of 6-7, the adrenal androgen hormones begin to increase, although most children show no obvious outward signs of the presence of these hormones in mid-childhood. The levels continue to rise throughout late childhood and adolescence. These adrenal hormones contribute to acne and the development of pubic and underarm hair as puberty progresses. Estrogen is made by the ovaries in girls and testosterone is made by the testes in boys. Both boys and girls make testosterone and estrogen, but girls make much more estrogen and boys much more testosterone. Both estrogen and testosterone contribute to growth in height. Estrogen increases the growth of bones but also causes the growth plates in the bones to close, which causes growth in height to stop gradually after the pubertal growth spurt. Estrogen also causes breasts to grow and bones to get denser by helping calcium absorption. In boys, testosterone causes increased growth in height, enlargement of the penis, increasing body and facial hair, and increased muscle development in both size and strength. Around the ages of 18-20, when boys stop growing, they may find that their body fat increases and they can become overweight if they exercise less and continue to eat the large amounts of food and take the large doses of insulin that they needed during their growth spurt a few years earlier.

In the normal population, there is a great deal of variation in growth in height. Just look at your own family. Some individuals grow more than others during childhood and puberty. Multiple genes contribute to growth in height, so that although height is genetically based, within one family there may be some shorter and some taller individuals, all of whom are growing normally for their particular set of genetic instructions. Growth charts in height, weight, and body mass index (weight for height) are very useful for pediatricians and diabetes specialists in evaluating growth. A normal pattern of growth occurs when a child grows along the same height or weight percentile, whereas it is more of a concern when a child's growth pattern changes and slows in height or weight gain. Your child with diabetes will usually see his or her diabetes team every 3 months. Height and weight and body mass index are plotted on the growth chart at each visit, as assessing growth is a very important part of diabetes care.

Menstrual Cycles

It is common for girls with diabetes to have irregular menstrual cycles or periods. A normal ovulatory menstrual cycle in which one egg ripens lasts between 25-45 days. Periods will normally last 7 days or less. Many woman experience menstrual cramps and feel pain in the lower abdomen, lower back, or upper legs on the first day of the period. This is caused by hormones called prostaglandins which cause the uterus, which contains muscle, to contract. In addition, some girls feel faint or have nausea, vomiting, or diarrhea on the first day of the period. These symptoms are usually relieved by medications like ibuprofen or naproxen. In some cases of more severe cramps, oral contraceptives containing estrogen and progestin may be used to treat these symptoms. These medications can be used by girls with diabetes. In the first two years after periods start, about half of teen girls have irregular cycles. If periods come more often than every 25 days, counting the first day of one period to the first day of the next period, or if periods last longer than 7 days, this is considered excessive bleeding. This pattern of frequent prolonged periods is relatively common in early adolescence and may require evaluation and treatment with medroxyprogesterone (Provera) or oral contraceptives for a few months. Occasionally, hereditary clotting disorders present as heavy bleeding with the start of menstrual cycles. By 5 years after the onset of menstrual cycles, about 5-10% of women will have irregular periods. If your teen has not had a period for 3 months, she should discuss this with her healthcare provider. Teens with poorly controlled diabetes very often have infrequent and irregular periods.

Causes of Irregular Periods

Evaluation of very irregular or infrequent periods in young women with diabetes includes a careful history and a general physical exam looking for signs of hormone imbalance. This exam may include a review of the following items:

- Thyroid — looking for signs of an underactive or overactive thyroid
- Androgen excess — looking for increased body hair or acne
- The breasts — looking for signs of hormonal imbalance
- Sometimes a pelvic exam or pelvic ultrasound
- Hormone levels by blood test
- A urine or blood pregnancy test

Women who are quite thin and who are intensely involved in athletic activities, such as distance running, can sometimes stop having periods as their estrogen levels drop due to the combination of inadequate nutrition, stress, and prolonged daily exercise. Very poor diabetes control can also result in a low estrogen state. A simple inspection of the outside of the vaginal area can help the healthcare provider in assessing whether the young woman is making estrogen normally. The medication medroxyprogesterone (Provera) is sometimes given for 10 days to bring on a period. It can be helpful to keep a calendar recording the dates of periods if they are irregular.

One of the most common causes of irregular periods in young women is polycystic ovary syndrome (PCOS). Young women with this pattern often have gradually increasing body hair on their abdomen and increasing hair on their face. They often have increased problems with acne and may gain weight easily. Some women have darkening and thickening of the skin on the back of their neck and under their arms. This is called *acanthosis nigricans* and is a sign of insulin resistance. Recent studies have found an increased percentage of young adult women with type 1 diabetes who have polycystic ovary syndrome compared to the general population. Type 2 diabetes is very commonly associated with polycystic ovary syndrome as well. An oral medication called metformin and oral contraceptives are commonly used to treat polycystic ovary syndrome. Antiandrogens such as spironolactone are sometimes added if increased body hair continues to be an issue despite ongoing treatment with oral contraceptives which lower the levels of androgen (testosterone like) hormones.

Preventing Unplanned Pregnancy and Transmitted Infections

Kids today are exposed to a lot of information, including information about sexuality. Your kids need someone to help filter a lot of information, answer questions and provide support, as physically and emotionally they develop that wonderful but often confusing array of sexual feelings. Families, and individuals within families, have different beliefs and values in this area. You need to decide when and how age-appropriate discussions occur with your child about sex, pregnancy, and sexually transmitted diseases.

Concerns for Women

Women with diabetes need to plan their pregnancies. Any teen who is concerned about a delayed period deserves a confidential discussion with her healthcare provider, since it is vital to diagnose a pregnancy without delay. It is important for the diabetes care provider to have discussions with your daughter early in her teen years about the significance of planning ahead for pregnancy, long before this becomes an immediate concern for her. It can be helpful to begin these discussions early in adolescence, when your daughter is receiving the series of 3 vaccines to decrease the risk of human papilloma virus in later life. At around this age, the diabetes care provider may discuss the importance of maintaining confidentiality and privacy with your teen. Some teens may be reluctant to discuss their concerns about pregnancy and sexually transmitted diseases with their parents. It is important that they know they can get reliable information on confidential concerns from their healthcare team.

Diabetes care providers and adolescent healthcare providers encourage teens to postpone sexual intercourse until they are mature young adults in a committed, caring relationship. During early adolescence, your diabetes provider may begin to spend a few minutes during the visit talking to your teen alone. The diabetes team tries hard to help young women with diabetes postpone sexual relations and avoid pregnancy in adolescence, since unplanned pregnancies in teens with diabetes are risky for the young mother as well as for her developing fetus.

When young women with diabetes plan a pregnancy as an adult, prior to the start of pregnancy they should first get their blood glucoses in superb control with goals of:

- Pre-meal blood glucose levels of 60-100 mg/dL
- Post-meal blood glucose levels of under 120 mg/dL

They will need help with frequent (weekly) medical visits during pregnancy to manage changing insulin requirements as the pregnancy progresses. They should be reassured that they can expect to have a healthy baby when they are ready to do all of the work required to manage a pregnancy with diabetes as an adult. Poor control of diabetes during pregnancy is associated with increased risks of miscarriage, birth defects, ketoacidosis, and severe hypoglycemic events. If women decide to be sexually active, they need effective contraception to avoid unplanned pregnancy. This would usually include a barrier method (condoms) to reduce the risk of sexually transmitted infection, and oral contraceptives. If diabetes control is poor, or if there are other contraindications to estrogen, progestin-only minipills or depot formulation of medroxyprogesterone (Depot Provera) may be preferred to estrogen-containing pills; however, oral contraceptives are a better health choice than an unplanned pregnancy if the diabetes is in poor control. Young women who have poor diabetes control need to remember that they can get pregnant even if they only have a few periods a year. Effective contraception is especially essential for young women at risk for pregnancy who have poor diabetes control. Young women should know that if they do have a single episode of unprotected sexual intercourse, immediate use (within 72 hours of intercourse) of Plan B (levonorgestrel) tablets is an option to decrease the risk of pregnancy. This medication is safe even for women with poorly controlled diabetes.

Aside from pregnancy, another area of concern for adolescent girls with diabetes is the occurrence of vaginal yeast infections. Women with frequent high blood glucoses can develop vaginal yeast infections more commonly than women without diabetes. Symptoms are itching and irritation of the vaginal opening, and/or a white lumpy vaginal discharge. Yeast infections can be treated with creams or suppositories available over the counter, or with a pill called fluconazole (Diflucan). Since other causes of vaginitis, some due to sexually transmitted infections, can present with similar symptoms, a young woman who thinks she has a yeast infection should be seen by her medical provider for a simple vaginal exam. Girls and women can also develop bacterial infections of the bladder known as urinary tract infections. These can present with urinary frequency, an urgency and painful urination. Urinary tract infections can occur more frequently when women have vaginal sexual intercourse. A woman who has symptoms of a urinary tract infection should see her healthcare provider promptly for a urine culture and antibiotics.

Concerns for Men

Males who decide to be sexually active should use condoms to decrease their risk of acquiring a sexually transmitted infection and to decrease their female partner's chance of becoming pregnant. Boys with diabetes may have concerns that they will have difficulty with impotence at some point during their life. Chronically elevated blood glucoses over many years can damage the small blood vessels of the penis causing difficulty achieving erections in some adult men with long-term diabetes. This is not an immediate problem for teens. Hypoglycemia (a low blood glucose), can cause temporary difficulty in having an erection. Teen boys often worry that this is the start of a more serious problem, and can be reassured that this is a normal and a temporary result of a low blood glucose level. Males with diabetes can develop fungal infections in the groin area more commonly if they have frequent high blood glucoses. The rash is itchy and the skin is red. These fungal infections (jock itch) can be treated with over the counter antifungal creams such as clortrimazole (Lotrimin) or tolnaftate (Tinactin, Ting). Pain on urination or a penile discharge should be a reason for seeking prompt medical attention as this could be a symptom of a sexually transmitted infection.

Team Care for Teens with Diabetes

Teens with diabetes need to have both a diabetes care provider with whom they feel comfortable talking and a primary care provider who is comfortable addressing adolescent health issues. Ideally, the diabetes care team and the primary adolescent healthcare providers should communicate and work together to address your teen's health concerns as completely as possible. As your child becomes a teen, he or she will begin to learn to use the healthcare team independently as a resource in getting advice for medical issues. This is an important step in helping your teen to manage diabetes care and overall health as an emerging adult.

Resources

Web sites:

- Growth Chart: www.brightfutures.org
- American Diabetes Association: www.diabetes.org
- JDRF: www.jdrf.org

13

Diabetes and Family Issues

When a child or teenager is diagnosed with diabetes, the whole family is affected. Children with diabetes need emotional support from parents and siblings, and they also require a great deal of practical support. Parents need support, too! Given the number of tasks that need to be completed every day, family teamwork is essential. This chapter provides tips that we hope you will find helpful as you and your family navigate life with diabetes.

Diabetes isn't easy, and the challenges change over time. Children, preteens, and teenagers each have specific concerns that might make certain aspects of diabetes more difficult. Young children cannot understand the complicated medical concepts of diabetes and may focus on the fear or discomfort associated with injections, whereas teens may be more sensitive to how diabetes makes them different from their peers. The length of time a child or teenager has had diabetes may also influence how challenging it feels. Sometimes young people adjust to diabetes fairly quickly, only to struggle with diabetes burnout further down the road; other times, the initial adjustment takes longer but diabetes management goes smoothly for quite some time after diagnosis. Parents often ask what to expect, but the fact is there is no typical path. What we do know is that diabetes challenges will feel less intense at some times and more intense at others. It's important to remember that your child's healthcare team has helped many families cope with the stresses of diabetes, and many families have worked to find creative solutions to typical diabetes challenges. With good communication, patience, teamwork, and advice from professionals and other families, your child and family can thrive.

Realistic Expectations

As you cope with diabetes, it is important to have realistic expectations. You should not expect perfect blood glucose values — in fact, we like to eliminate the word perfect from the diabetes vocabulary. It is impossible to achieve perfect blood glucose control with the tools and technology that are currently available. Even when your child follows his or her diabetes plan exactly, there will still be times when he or she does not get the expected results. For example, you might see a higher blood glucose number than usual because your child is coming down with a cold, even though he or she is not showing cold symptoms yet. These limitations can be hard for parents to accept, because you want to be able to have complete control over keeping your child healthy. There is a great deal you can do to ensure that your child has a long, healthy life — and remember that technology is always improving — but it is still important to have realistic goals.

Also remember that it is virtually impossible for anyone to achieve perfect adherence to a diabetes plan all the time. Life is not that predictable, and human beings aren't perfect. Aim to do the best you can do. Follow instructions as closely as you can, and when you have a difficult day, know that you will have a chance to start over tomorrow. Whenever you find that you are struggling with managing your child's diabetes, talk to your child's healthcare team. They may have some ideas that could help you.

How the Diagnosis of Diabetes Affects the Family

One of the hardest periods for families is at the time of diagnosis. The diagnosis usually comes as a shock. Unfortunately, diabetes does not allow you time to adjust to the news before you have to jump right into learning a tremendous amount of new information and many new skills. Learning how to take care of diabetes is a big job and can be overwhelming, plus you are in the midst of the emotional turmoil that usually comes with diagnosis. At the beginning, it is normal to feel consumed by diabetes. Many parents find it reminiscent of when they first brought their child home. The sense of responsibility, the fear and anxiety about your child's well-being, the pressure of wanting to do everything exactly right, and the fear of making a mistake are all normal reactions. Just as taking care of a child feels more manageable once you have had time to learn, practice, and adjust, taking care of diabetes will also become part of your daily life. Tasks that once seemed complicated and intimidating will become routine.

Finding the New "Normal"

Once your family has had some time to adjust to the information and new routines that come with a diagnosis of diabetes, it is important to establish a new sense of normal as soon as possible. Whenever possible, diabetes care should be adapted to fit your child's lifestyle, rather than your child's life revolving around diabetes. We believe that diabetes should not define who your child is, so we do not like to label children as diabetics. Children with diabetes are children first, and they need to know that they should try to do everything they would have done if they had not been diagnosed with diabetes. For example, if your child played soccer before diagnosis, he or she should continue to play soccer after diagnosis. Or, if cupcakes were a normal part of birthday parties before diabetes, then your child should still be able to have a cupcake at a party. Your child's healthcare team can help you adapt his or her diabetes regimen to allow for these activities.

It is also important to examine how diabetes is impacting the entire family, and to check on whether diabetes is dominating family life. Some families find that diabetes has taken over their lives, especially in the period just after diagnosis. As a parent, it can be very difficult to shift your focus away from diabetes because you are so concerned about your child's health and safety. But when diabetes begins to define the parent-child relationship, it may be very difficult for both the parent and the child. For example, we hear from many children and teens that the first question they're asked when they come home from school is not, "How was your day?" but rather "What was your blood glucose?" or "Have you checked?". This is frustrating for kids, and it often sets the stage for conflict related to diabetes. We suggest trying to treat your child with diabetes the same way you treated your child before he or she was diagnosed, and the same way you treat your other children without diabetes. We also suggest talking about the same things you talked about before your child was diagnosed with diabetes. So in the example above, try asking your child about his or her day at school before asking about diabetes. This approach may help your child feel more patient when discussions do need to focus on diabetes.

Sibling Issues

Although other children in the family may not be directly involved in diabetes care, they too are affected by diabetes. Due to the energy and focus that diabetes management requires, other children in the family may feel left out, especially at the time of diagnosis. Siblings may feel jealous of all of the attention that is being directed at the child with diabetes — in much the same way that children may struggle with the birth of a new sibling. Siblings may also be confused and scared by what is happening, and they may have worries about whether their brother or sister is going to be okay. Many siblings worry about whether they too will get diabetes. A diabetes diagnosis may also lead families to change what foods are kept in the house, or to change other family routines, such as the timing of meals or snacks. These changes can be difficult for siblings. We recommend that you provide support and information to the other children in the family and make sure that they get individual attention just as they did before diabetes. Some siblings want to help their brother or sister with diabetes and your healthcare team can help you find age-appropriate ways for them to be involved. Other times, siblings do not want to be involved. We suggest that you do not force them to participate in diabetes care. Remember that siblings do not stop acting like siblings just because of diabetes! Brothers and sisters may still annoy each other and squabble sometimes, and this can actually be a sign that things are returning to normal. You may wish to watch for teasing related to diabetes, however, and to speak to your children about what is and is not acceptable behavior in your family.

Sharing Responsibility for Diabetes

Given the number of daily tasks involved in diabetes management, it is normal for everyone in the family to feel burned out from diabetes from time to time. Unfortunately there is no break from diabetes, which is why sharing diabetes tasks is so important. We encourage each member of the family to keep tabs on how he or she is feeling so that the balance of responsibility can be shifted as needed. In two-parent families, job responsibilities or other factors may lead one parent to assume more responsibility for child care and diabetes care. One parent may also be more comfortable with medical tasks or diabetes calculations in the beginning, so he or she may naturally fall into the role of primary diabetes caretaker. Some parents recognize that they like to be in control and tell us that it is hard to learn to share diabetes responsibility with their partners, and other parents may feel left out or more anxious about diabetes care. Nonetheless, it is important for both parents to be involved and to shift responsibility back and forth so that no one caregiver becomes too overburdened or too left out. Family members or babysitters should also be trained to perform diabetes tasks so that couples can take time for themselves. The extra responsibility of diabetes can be stressful for marriages and families, and it is important to seek support if you need it. Your children will benefit by your taking care of yourself.

For single parents, it is important to find other adults who can learn about diabetes and help give you a break. Extended family members and friends may be willing to come to medical appointments to learn about diabetes care. Organizations like the American Diabetes Association (ADA) and the Juvenile Diabetes Research Foundation (JDRF) can also be good sources of support and information. You may be able to meet another family in your area that is affected by diabetes, and you can potentially help each other with child care.

It is likely that your healthcare team has worked with many different types of families, and they can help you figure out how to get the support you need. It is important to seek advice when there are any family transitions, such as a separation, a divorce, or a new marriage, as these events often require families to learn new ways of communicating about and sharing responsibility for diabetes tasks.

It is also important to monitor your child's level of responsibility for diabetes care, as his or her needs may change over time. There is no age at which your child or teen should assume the full responsibility for taking care of his or her diabetes. Just as responsibility for diabetes care can lead to parent or caretaker burnout, diabetes can also lead to burnout in children and teens. In younger children, burnout can take the form of increased frustration with diabetes tasks, reduced cooperation or general signs of sadness or anger. It works well to allow young children to have choices versus responsibility. Choice of a site for a shot or pump, a finger for a finger-stick, or the choice between salad and a cooked vegetable provides personal power over diabetes self-management tasks. Older children and teenagers who have been carrying a significant share of the responsibility for their diabetes management may start to pay less attention to diabetes care because they are burned out or because they simply have other priorities, and they may need parents to step in and share or resume responsibility for diabetes tasks. Just because children or teenagers *can* perform management tasks doesn't mean they *should have to* all the time. We find that increasing parental involvement works best when it is not presented as a punishment or a sign that the child or teen has failed to take care of him- or herself. Instead, explain to your child that it is important to work as a team and that you would like to offer more support. Some children and teens may be especially likely to expect too much of themselves and be hesitant to ask for help, because they put pressure on themselves to be independent and responsible. For this reason, it is important for parents to check in with children and teens periodically to see if diabetes has become too burdensome.

Lastly, it is important to consider the impact of diabetes responsibility sharing on the parent-child relationship. When children are young, it is typical for parents to be very involved in their daily activities and to assume the majority of responsibility for most caretaking tasks. In families affected by diabetes, the need for medical management requires parents to remain more intimately involved with their child's daily routines than they normally would as children get older. For example, parents may need to know about everything their fourth grader with diabetes eats, when this would not be the case for a fourth grader without diabetes. The need for parent involvement with diabetes extends far into the teenage years, and this can clash with teenagers' desire for greater independence. This can set the stage for conflict. Communication with your healthcare team about how to balance the need for diabetes-related involvement with your child's growing need for independence can be helpful. Small interventions, such as leaving a blood glucose meter on the kitchen counter so that parents can check blood glucose values without having to bother their teenager, can ease tension and allow for continued parent involvement that is more comfortable for your teen. A switch to this type of nonverbal communication can eliminate hotspots that may turn into an argument. It is clear that young people with diabetes continue to benefit from parental involvement even into early adulthood, so make sure to continue to work as a team to determine the best ways for parents to remain involved.

Healthy Communication

Positive communication is another critical component of successful diabetes management. Many children naturally want to please their parents, and this applies to diabetes as well. Try to think about how your family communicates about diabetes-specific issues. If your child's blood glucose is in the 100's, you may find yourself telling your child that is a good number and you may act very excited. Conversely, if your child's blood glucose is in the 300's, you may find yourself becoming more negative and having a more serious look on your face. This can lead children with diabetes to learn that telling their parents that their blood glucose is 122, even if it is 322, will make their parents happy or allow them to avoid feeling like they are in trouble. Yet with inaccurate information, parents cannot make accurate decisions about diabetes care. This is why it is so important to pay attention to your language. Table 13-1 shows words you can use to encourage positive communication about diabetes. It is hard for many parents not to have an emotional reaction to individual meter readings or to feel like the number is a grade on a test,

Table 13-1. Words to Encourage Positive Communication about Diabetes

Instead of saying...	Try saying...
Please *test* your blood glucose.	Please *check* your blood glucose.
That is a *good* blood glucose number.	That blood glucose is *in range.*
That is a *bad* blood glucose number.	The blood glucose number is *high* so I am going to give you some extra insulin.
Good job with that blood glucose number!	I am so glad you checked your blood glucose. You are trying hard to take care of your diabetes!
What did you eat to make your blood glucose so high? Have you been eating candy?	Let's watch over the next few days to see if your blood glucose is high at this time each day.

but we encourage families to think of the blood glucose meter as if it's a GPS device that always provides good information, because it tells you where you are and what direction you need to go next. A low number might mean a child needs juice or a snack, and a high number might mean that a child needs more insulin. This is also an important lesson for your child to learn for when he or she will be in charge of diabetes management tasks.

In addition to focusing on language, try to create an environment where your child feels comfortable telling you if he or she had an extra snack or missed a blood glucose check or forgot an insulin dose. Children and teenagers are less likely to reveal why the blood glucose may be high if they are worried that their parents will become disappointed or angry; if you create an environment where your child or teen can be honest with you about his or her struggles with diabetes management, then you can be proactive, problem-solve together, and come up with solutions as a team. Setting this tone for family life in general, and diabetes in particular, will make life much more pleasant.

Once you have created an environment where honest communication is possible, it is important to listen. It may be difficult for you to understand how your teen could forget to check his or her blood glucose at a certain time of day, but he or she may be able to help you understand why something got missed. Perhaps he or she is focused on getting to lunch on time and does not want to go to the nurse's office. You may be frustrated that your child ate unhealthy snacks at a friend's house, but it may be that he or she was shy about asking for healthier snacks, and didn't want to feel different from friends. If your child does not tell you these things, then you cannot come up with strategies to help.

Some families find it helpful to set aside a specific time each week when they can talk about diabetes. For example, on Sunday evenings you may want to check in with your child and ask how he or she is doing and what has been hard about having diabetes. You may be surprised to hear the answers. This might be a great time to review his or her meter or logbook. Setting aside a special time to talk also helps to remind parents to spend the rest of the week focusing on issues other than diabetes.

Listening to your child will also help you avoid misguided helping. Most adults have had the experience of a family member or friend offering advice that is intended to be helpful but is actually upsetting or counterproductive, especially at the time of diagnosis. Miscarried helping occurs when a well-meaning individual is trying to help the child with diabetes, but this help does not come across as supportive. Instead, the child ends up feeling resentful or criticized. For example, parents might decide to stop reminding their child to do blood glucose checks or to take insulin so that their child can learn to do this on his or her own. Parents may think they are being helpful by pulling back and not giving diabetes reminders, but the child may feel neglected instead and stop performing diabetes tasks to get back at his or her parents for withdrawing their support.

We encourage you to avoid making assumptions about how your child is feeling, why he or she is or is not following through with certain diabetes tasks, and how you can help. It is always essential to ask. Sometimes kids don't check their blood glucose because they forget. In this case, they might appreciate a reminder. Other times, they may not check because they are feeling burned out and are avoiding anything that makes them think about diabetes. In this case, the child or teen would need a different kind of support. Simply stated, you are the parent and are responsible for your child with diabetes receiving the best care, time, effort and concern you can provide. There will be roadblocks at ages and stages as your child grows and develops. Your healthcare team, or a counselor who is experienced in working with families, can help parents and children express themselves and find ways to work together more effectively so that the family can find solutions that will work for everyone. Diabetes web sites can be another helpful source of tips and solutions that have worked for other families. Several diabetes web sites are included in the resource list at the end of this chapter.

Finally, it is important to be mindful of which diabetes-related conversations are appropriate for the whole family, which should occur with your child with diabetes, and which issues should be restricted to adult discussions. Younger children who overhear conversations related to diabetes issues cannot fully understand and can become anxious. Even the word diabetes may be anxiety-provoking for young children, who sometimes hear DIE-abetes. Children and adults may have questions about diabetes risks and complications, particularly at the time of diagnosis. It can be helpful to ask your child or teen if he or she has any fears so that you and your child's healthcare team can provide accurate information. It may also be important to ask relatives or family friends about any fears or concerns they may have about your child's diabetes. Have these conversations when your child is not present. Family members or friends may have had unfortunate outcomes themselves from diabetes or know someone else who struggled with diabetes, and this may cause them to worry about your child or even to express these concerns to your child. Keep in mind that these family members or friends remember stories about people who managed diabetes years before today's tools and technologies were available, therefore your child can expect different outcomes with careful management. (Detailed information on long-term complications is provided in Chapter 16: Long-Term Complications and Co-Morbidities.)

For children and teens of all ages, we counsel that you do not threaten them with fears about long-term diabetes-related complications. It is very normal for parents to worry about long-term complications, but it is not normal for children and teens to worry about their long-term health. We have had several parents ask us to try and scare their child or teen about what will happen to them if they do not take care of themselves, but we do not find this helpful. In fact, it may make things worse, as fear or a sense of hopelessness can cause children and teens to avoid thinking about diabetes altogether and to stop paying attention to diabetes tasks. Young people are motivated by what will happen in the present rather than the future, so try not to use scare tactics about long-term diabetes complications to motivate your child to take care of him- or herself. Instead, try to focus on priorities and goals that are important to your child. For example, if your child is an athlete, help her make the connection between stable blood glucose levels and optimal sports performance. If your child is focused on academics, emphasize that having in-range blood glucose values may help him perform best in school.

Compromise

Balancing good communication and listening is necessary for successful diabetes management, and so is compromise. Children and parents may have different goals, concerns, and motivations when it comes to taking care of diabetes. It is easier to find solutions that work for everyone when each person's unique point of view is taken into account. For parents,

Table 13-2. Parent versus Youth Priorities

Parents' Priorities	Youth Priorities
• Diabetes care • Following healthcare instructions • Making healthy decisions	• Age-appropriate concerns like – Schoolwork – Friends – Music or sports – Fitting in • Diabetes can – Feel like a nuisance that interrupts daily activities – Feel like a heavy burden that makes one feel different or embarrassed

both short-term safety and long-term health are usually primary concerns. For children and teens, health is less of a focus. Diabetes goals are easiest to achieve with strategies that honor the priorities of both parents and children. Table 13-2 presents a comparison of parent and youth priorities.

Important questions to ask when working toward good communication and compromise include:

- What do I need and want?
- What does my child need and want?
- What parts of this situation cannot be changed?
- What parts of this situation are flexible?
- Is there a solution that will accommodate everyone's needs and wants?
- How can we come up with a solution that everyone is comfortable with?

Let's take the example given earlier, when we reviewed the importance of good communication. Say your child is missing blood glucose checks at school. As a parent, you are concerned that he or she may not get an adequate insulin dose without a blood glucose check. This is frustrating because you are worried about his or her glycemic control and safety, and it's hard to understand why he or she would fail to complete a quick and simple check when it is so important. Your child, on the other hand, is focused on getting to lunch in a hurry so that he or she can find a good seat and sit with friends. If your child goes to the school nurse's office to check his or her blood glucose, then there may not be any seats left by the time he or she gets to the cafeteria. Solving this problem requires finding a solution that addresses your needs and your child's needs, so that you know your child is getting the right amount of insulin and will get to the cafeteria at the same time as the other students. To solve the problem, you could speak with your child's school to find an alternate strategy. This might mean allowing your child to leave class a few minutes early to check his or her blood glucose before going to lunch. In some states, children with diabetes are allowed to check their blood glucose anywhere in the school, so some children may just check their blood glucose in their classroom or in the cafeteria.

You might be surprised at the creative solutions your family can come up with if you open the lines of communication about diabetes. When children and teens are asked the simple question, "What would make this easier?", they are often able to describe simple, specific strategies that will make diabetes care a little more manageable for them but would require only minimal compromise from parents. For example, many children do not like it when diabetes interrupts their activities. A simple change, such as going to where your child is playing when it is time for an injection versus calling him to come to where you are, can make a big difference.

Remember, it may be helpful to give your child choices whenever possible, because there are so many aspects of diabetes that do not allow for choice.

- For blood glucose checks, allow your child to choose which finger.
- For insulin administration, allow your child to choose from various injection sites (as approved by your child's healthcare team).
- For snacking, offer your child a choice of 2 or 3 healthy snacks and let him choose which snack he wants.

All of these examples allow your child to feel like he has more control while still ensuring optimal diabetes management.

Setting Limits

Even with an emphasis on good communication and compromise, sometimes your child or teen may have difficulty cooperating with diabetes tasks or following the prescribed medical regimen. This is to be expected. It is difficult for anyone, of any age, to cope with a chronic medical condition and to follow a daily routine. For this reason, we encourage parents to view diabetes tasks as separate from other responsibilities and to use different parenting techniques to address any problems that may arise. Failure to complete diabetes tasks is not the same as failure to complete homework or household chores, and we believe that punishment is not an effective means of addressing diabetes-related challenges. Instead, it is important to problem-solve with your child or teen and to avoid reactions that will make him or her feel ashamed, blamed, or guilty.

For parents who are focused on instilling a sense of responsibility in their children, this is often a confusing concept. Many parents feel that if their child does something wrong, then there should be a consequence. For example, if a teenager does not perform diabetes management tasks after school, then a parent may feel that he or she should not be allowed to go out with friends. We believe that it is normal for children and teens to have trouble with certain diabetes tasks, so children and teens who are struggling with their diabetes care need help, not punishment.

Another common challenge for parents of children with diabetes is how to set limits. You wish that you could make diabetes go away and it is difficult to see your child live with the inconveniences and discomfort of some diabetes regimens. You may even feel responsible for the diagnosis, but no one caused diabetes. You may find yourself wanting to indulge your child or wanting to reduce other demands and expectations — such as household chores — in order to compensate or make up for the child having diabetes. This is a natural impulse, but we have found that children and teens are more successful when they have the same rules, limits and responsibilities that they would have had if they had not been diagnosed with diabetes. Limits and rules reinforce the idea that they are normal kids who happen to have a medical condition.

Using Rewards

Many families have had success using the reward system for diabetes tasks. As discussed earlier, children typically want to please their parents. They also feel good when they accomplish a task. Reward systems differ from bribes in that children earn a reward as a direct result of a specific behavior, much as an adult might buy a new pair of jeans after working hard to lose weight. Since you are trying to encourage your child to cooperate with diabetes tasks and want to promote feelings of accomplishment, it is important to keep goals small and achievable so that your child can succeed. If a goal is too difficult, your child might end up feeling frustrated or demoralized. Small successes will lead to good feelings and more success, which allows for positive momentum. It can also be helpful to target one behavior at a time, such as wearing a diabetes identification bracelet every day, before adding additional goals. For younger children, sticker charts can be a very effective means of encouraging cooperation with diabetes tasks. Parents are often amazed at how quickly they can see improvement in their child's behavior or his or her willingness to try something new. For example, if your child is nervous about using a new injection site, you could give your child a sticker each time that he or she uses the new site. Each sticker is a small reward, and when your child has earned a predetermined number of stickers he or she can earn a small prize. This prize does not have to be a material item. It might be an extra bedtime story or time set aside for an activity with a parent.

For older children and teens, a sticker chart might be replaced with a check-off chart that works in much the same way. For example, if your teen has not been checking his or her blood glucose after school and then is able to check his or her blood glucose after school for 5 straight days, then he or she could earn a reward. You and your child or teen can come up with reasonable rewards or incentives that are motivating for him or her, such as extra time with the family or friends, movie passes, or other small items. Goal charts allow children and families to see how hard they are working to manage diabetes. Ask your healthcare team to help you develop a positive rewards program tailored to your child's interests and goals.

Family Teamwork

A common theme of this book is the focus on family teamwork. From the moment that your child is diagnosed with diabetes, it is important to stress to your child that regardless of his or her age, you will be taking care of diabetes together. Several parents have asked us at what age their child should start checking their own blood glucose, taking their own injections or insulin boluses or learning how to count carbohydrates. We have learned through both research and clinical experience that there is not a specific age at which children with diabetes should become independent with diabetes tasks. Instead, we stress the importance of ongoing family support at all stages of a child's development. So even if you think your child is old enough to learn how to draw up an insulin dose or give an injection, we promote parents to assume responsibility for these tasks for as long as possible and to allow children and teens to let you know when they would like more responsibility.

There are two reasons why we think parents should be in charge of diabetes tasks as long as possible. First, family teamwork is one of the best ways to prevent your child from feeling burned out from diabetes. Diabetes is a lifelong disease, so the more you help your child with diabetes now, the less burdened he or she may feel in the future. Second, family teamwork is also one of the best strategies for helping your child achieve optimal glycemic control. When children or teens take over more diabetes responsibilities, it is very common for them to forget a blood glucose check or insulin dose, to stop rotating injections or pump sites or to underestimate the amount of carbohydrates they are consuming. Children and teens may also be more apt to start eating without taking their insulin, only to remember an hour or two later when their blood glucose has already spiked. Children and teens also may not want to take the time to look over blood glucose patterns. Therefore, family teamwork can help in these areas and becomes necessary for successful diabetes management.

Eventually you may want your child or teen to take over some diabetes management tasks. However, one should not force a child or teen to self-manage diabetes. Some children or teens can take over some simple diabetes management tasks gradually. For example, if your teen wants to go to a sleepover but does not want you to come over to give him or her the bedtime insulin injection, then your teen might be motivated to learn how to self-inject in order to go to a friend's house. In this situation, we still encourage the parent to give the teen bedtime insulin when he or she is at home, but the teen may continue to give injections at a friend's house. Do not worry if you know another child with diabetes who is the same age as your child and giving him- or herself injections. Every child and teen is different. If you have any questions about whether your child or teen has too much or too little diabetes-specific responsibility, please discuss this issue with your child's healthcare team.

A Final Ingredient — Using Humor

Just as every child and teen is unique, every family with diabetes is unique. This chapter has outlined general guidelines for communication and family teamwork and we hope you will be able to adapt many of the concepts to specific situations you face in your own family. A final critical ingredient for successful family management of diabetes is a sense of humor. Diabetes can be stressful, and family members sometimes get frustrated or irritated with one another. Humor can help defuse certain tense situations and help family members stay calm. Humor will also help put your child at ease. The more fun you have together as a family, the more energy you will have to work together as a team and manage diabetes.

References and Resources

Anderson BJ, Coyne JC. "Miscarried helping" in the interactions between chronically ill children and their parents. In: Johnson JH, Johnson SB (Eds.), *Advances in Child Health Psychology*. Gainesville, FL: University of Florida Press, 1991:167-177.

Anderson BJ. The Home Team Advantage. *Diabetes Self Management.* September/October 1994; 55-59.

Anderson, B.J., Vangness, L., Connell, A., Butler, D., Goebel-Fabbri, A.E., & Laffel, L. Family conflict, adherence, and glycemic control in youth with short term duration type 1 diabetes. *Diabetic Medicine*. 2002;19, 635-642 .

Butler DA, Zuchlke JB, Tovar A, Volkening LK, Anderson BJ, Laffel LM. The impact of modifiable family factors on glycemic control among youth with type 1 diabetes. *Pediatric Diabetes*. 2008; 9(4 Pt 2):373-381.

Laffel, L., Vangness, L., Connell, A., Goebel-Fabbri, A., Butler, D., & Anderson, B. J. Impact of ambulatory, family-focused teamwork intervention on glycemic control in youth with type 1 diabetes. *Journal of Pediatrics*. 2003;142, 409-416.

Shiller VM, Schneider MF, Matthews B. *Rewards for Kids!: Ready-to-Use Charts & Activities for Positive Parenting*. Washington, DC: American Psychological Association, 2003.

Web sites:

- The Joslin Diabetes Center: www.joslin.org
  - Joslin Diabetes Center Discussion Boards: http://forums.joslin.org/
- Children with Diabetes.com: www.childrenwithdiabetes.com
- American Diabetes Association (ADA): www.diabetes.org
  - ADA online community for children and teens: http://tracker.diabetes.org/
- Juvenile Diabetes Research Foundation (JDRF) International: www.jdrf.org
  - Online diabetes community created by JDRF: juvenation.org

14

Behavioral and Psychological Pitfalls — Prevention and Early Intervention

Families experience certain challenges when their child has diabetes. It is important to tell your child's diabetes healthcare team when you are faced with obstacles or stressors that are having a negative impact on your child's diabetes control. Here are some common pitfalls that families living with diabetes experience during the pediatric years and some strategies to try if you are faced with any of these situations.

Pitfalls at Diagnosis

When your child is diagnosed with diabetes it can be very overwhelming, both physically and emotionally. Your child may have spent a few days in the hospital, or you may have received diabetes survival skills in an outpatient setting and had several medical providers teaching you how to manage your child's diabetes in a very short period of time.

A lot of parents are afraid to give their child an insulin injection or do a finger-stick for blood glucose monitoring. Even though this sounds extremely overwhelming, parents learn to overcome these fears so that they can keep their child healthy. We suggest that parents practice giving injections on a doll or insulin pillow. After you are comfortable giving injections on a doll or pillow, consider practicing on yourself or another caretaker using an injection with saline solution. Then, before you give your child an injection, try to relax. Consider taking a deep breath. If you are feeling scared, your child is going to pick up on your anxiety, so the more relaxed you are, the more relaxed your child will be. If you are living in a 2-parent home, or there are other adult caretakers in the home, make sure all parents/caretakers are comfortable giving injections. It is very common for one adult to assume more of the responsibility for injections after diagnosis, so we suggest that your child become comfortable with more than one person giving him or her an injection. For example, some families divide the injections up so that the same adult gives the morning injections each day and then another adult gives the evening injections.

If your child is very anxious around injection times and is fighting with you or screaming at you, you may want to try a few of these strategies:

- Try to minimize the amount of time it takes to give your child an injection. Prepare everything (for example, pre-fill the syringe) before calling your child for the injection or going to your child to give the injection.
- Try not to give your child an injection while in his or her bed, so that the bed remains a calming place in the house for your child. A lot of families say they give injections in the kitchen where they keep the diabetes supplies, and that this works well.
- Suggest that your child take a deep breath; or, if your child is younger, you may want to use a distraction technique such as blowing bubbles or a pinwheel. Relaxing your child by taking a few deep breathes may help make the injection feel less painful.
- Try not to restrain your child if possible, but consider trying more comfortable positions for him or her.

The insulin injection should be quick and just take a few minutes. If you are finding that insulin injections are taking a long time, and none of the above strategies are working, then we suggest that you talk to your child's diabetes healthcare team. Your team may have some other ideas to help you, like trying an automatic injector, using a syringe with a shorter needle, or trying an insulin pen.

Also, remember the suggestions that were mentioned in Chapter 13: Diabetes and Family Issues:

- Work with your diabetes healthcare team so that your child can participate in all of the activities that he or she participated in before being diagnosed with diabetes.
- Maintain the same rules and expectations that your child had before being diagnosed with diabetes; children with diabetes need the same rules and structure as children without diabetes.
- Do not forget to spend time with your other children without diabetes and check in with them to see how they are doing.

Dealing with Severe Hypoglycemia

Many parents fear that their child could have a severe low blood glucose. A lot of parents fear that it will happen during the middle of the night or when their child is away from home. Some parents even worry about what they would do if their child had a severe low blood glucose and they needed to give their child a glucagon injection (see Chapter 9: Hypoglycemia for more information on how to treat severe hypoglycemia). If you have had the unfortunate experience of witnessing your child have severe low blood glucose, you may have seen your child have a seizure or lose consciousness. This can be a very scary and frightening thing to observe; your child, on the other hand, will probably not remember what happened. This is why episodes of severe hypoglycemia can be more traumatic for the individuals that witness the episode than for the person with diabetes. It can be very difficult for parents to forget the image of their child's severe hypoglycemic event.

Some parents have such a fear of hypoglycemia that they tend to run their child's blood glucose higher than what is prescribed by the child's diabetes healthcare team. If you find yourself in this situation, it is important that you talk to your child's team so they can work with you around this issue. One strategy that the team may recommend is checking your child's blood glucose more often, because frequent blood glucose monitoring is one of the best strategies to prevent severe hypoglycemia. Your child's diabetes healthcare team may also recommend that you check your child's blood glucose in the middle of the night, especially if this is the time your child tends to have lows. If you find that you are still worrying about whether your child will have an episode of severe hypoglycemia, even with more frequent blood glucose monitoring, you may want to ask your child's team for a referral to a mental health counselor that is knowledgeable about diabetes.

Negative Communication Traps

Most families find that it can be difficult to talk about diabetes. Many families find themselves fighting about diabetes related issues from time to time. The most common period that diabetes conflict occurs is during adolescence. Some of the most common diabetes issues that families tend to fight about include:

- Blood glucose monitoring (*e.g.*, not checking before meals, sports, or driving, etc.)
- Insulin administration (*e.g.*, forgetting insulin shots or boluses)
- Forgetting diabetes supplies (*e.g.*, not carrying diabetes supplies to a friend's house or not wearing a diabetes ID)
- The child's meal plan (*e.g.*, eating too much junk food or frequent snacking)

Some children and teens also fight with their parents because they think their parents are constantly nagging them about diabetes. When you find yourself fighting about diabetes issues and are caught up in a vicious cycle of negative communication, think about what you are fighting about. Is there anything that you could stop asking or reminding your child about? For example, instead of always asking your child what his or her blood glucose was at school, ask your child to leave the meter on the kitchen counter and you can go through the meter memory instead. Or if you are fighting with your child because you think he or she is missing blood glucose checks or insulin, maybe he or she has taken on too much diabetes responsibility. Maybe you need to take over more diabetes tasks and start providing the morning and evening insulin again. If your child is on a pump, maybe you should be in charge of pump site changes. If you are working together with your child as a team, you may find that you fight less about diabetes issues. If these strategies do not work, you may want to consider meeting with a counselor that is knowledgeable about diabetes and adolescents.

Also remember these strategies that we discussed in Chapter 13:

- Make sure that you discuss non-diabetes issues. For example, ask your child about his or her day when they come home from school before you ask about his or her blood glucose value.
- Do not use fear tactics to motivate your child with diabetes even if you are really frustrated and worried. For example, if your teen is worried about his or her appearance, you may want to mention that better blood glucose control may help his or her skin, or hair and nail growth.
- If you learn that your child has been falsifying blood glucose data, do not call your child a cheater or a liar. Instead try to move on and reinforce that it is okay to tell you the correct blood glucose value and give your child positive reinforcement for the act of checking a blood glucose versus giving positive reinforcement for the actual blood glucose value. Blood glucose values need to be treated as information instead of like a test grade or a "good" or 'bad" number.

Diabetes Burnout

At some point, most individuals with diabetes experience diabetes burnout. It is also a common experience for family members of individuals with diabetes. People experience diabetes burnout when they feel completely overwhelmed with diabetes management tasks. Diabetes is a 24-hour-a-day condition with no break, so there is always something to think about. For example, you need to think about diabetes every time you eat, when you are active, when you feel that your blood glucose may be low or high, when you are sick, when you travel, or when there is a schedule change. Diabetes burnout also occurs when individuals feel frustrated with diabetes management. For example, you may be doing everything that your child's diabetes healthcare team tells you to do, but you will still see out of range blood glucose from time to time. Unfortunately, the tools we have available now are not perfect, so it is impossible to maintain in range blood glucose values all of the time. Therefore, many individuals and family members experience diabetes burnout at some time.

If you are wondering if your child or teen is experiencing diabetes burnout, some of the signs include:

- Missing blood glucose checks
- Missing insulin shots or insulin boluses
- Not carbohydrate counting or reading food labels
- Your child seems more irritable about diabetes management tasks
- Increasing conflict between you and your child

Some children or teens occasionally get burned out from their particular diabetes regimen. For example, if your child is taking multiple injections a day and is growing very tired of injections, then you may want to consider talking to your healthcare team about an insulin pump. On the other hand, your child may be burned out from using and wearing an insulin pump. Your child may be tired of having a device attached to him or her all the time and constantly disconnecting and reconnecting the pump because of sports or activities. When this happens, some children find it helpful to take a pump vacation or break from using the pump. If you think your child is burned out then talk to your child's diabetes healthcare team about the possibility of switching diabetes regimens.

There are also several things you can do to both prevent and treat diabetes burnout that have already been highlighted. Remember to:

- Maintain and increase family involvement in diabetes management tasks. The more parents are involved with day to day diabetes management tasks, the less of a chance that the child or teen will experience diabetes burnout.
- Maintain realistic goals and expectations. Your child's diabetes healthcare team should be able to help you determine realis-

tic goals and expectations for your child based on age and development.

- Do not expect perfection. Aim for doing the best that you can, while making sure that your child's quality of life is not negatively impacted.
- Find more support, which includes a diabetes healthcare team that is knowledgeable about pediatric diabetes issues. You may also want to meet with a mental health or family support specialist (*e.g.*, clinical social worker or psychologist), attend a parent group or support group, or use an online chat room or forum. Diabetes can be a very isolating disease; it may be helpful to talk to other parents who understand what you are going through. Your child's diabetes healthcare team may host parent groups or may suggest some groups in your local area, or provide online resources.
- Consider sending your child to diabetes camp. Children who attend diabetes camps can have a fun time, but also have the opportunity to meet other children with diabetes. Diabetes camps can also be a great break for parents because it gives you one or two weeks a year when you do not need to manage your child's diabetes. Some diabetes camps also offer family weekends, which is a great way to meet other families living with diabetes (see Chapter 15: Schools, Parties, Relatives, Travel, and Camp for more information about diabetes camps).

Surviving Adolescence

Adolescence can be a very challenging time for families for many reasons. Following the course of normal development, teens:

- Start to question their own identity and want to be unique but not too different from their peers.
- Have a sense of being invincible.
- Engage in risk taking behavior.

- Worry about the present and do not think much about the future.
- Start to break away from their parents, by rejecting parental values and becoming more autonomous.

Unfortunately, all of these common and normal adolescent developmental behaviors make diabetes control more challenging. Teens with diabetes:

- Tend to want to forget about diabetes because they are becoming more spontaneous and finding more interesting distractions.
- Take on more diabetes responsibility, as they are breaking away from their parents and spending more time with their friends.
- Take risks, seek independence, and seek peer support like their counterparts who do not have diabetes.

As a result, you may see your child's blood glucose control deteriorate during adolescence.

There are several things you can do to make adolescence a less challenging time. Some of these strategies we have already mentioned.

- Do not avoid your child's diabetes healthcare team. Be honest with your team and let them know the areas in which you and your child have been struggling.
- Stay involved and help your teen with as many diabetes tasks as he or she will allow. Problem-solve with your teen and negotiate ways for you to stay involved. Your teen may be doing all of his or her own shots or boluses, but maybe your teen would let you help with insulin dosing and administration. If your teen is on the pump, maybe he or she will let you be in charge of site changes. Or maybe your teen may agree for you to go through his or her meter each night and call your child's diabetes healthcare team when you start to notice a pattern of low or high blood glucose values.

- Focus on all of the things that your teen is doing well versus what your teen is *not* doing. Praise your teen for all of the blood glucose checks and insulin shots or boluses that he or she does remember. If you are positive about what your teen is doing well with their diabetes, then your teen may be more honest with you about what issues he or she is struggling with.

You also may be worried about whether your teen is experimenting with drugs or alcohol. It is common for teens with or without diabetes to feel peer pressure to experiment. Some teens also use drugs or alcohol to self medicate because they are feeling overwhelmed with their lives or they may be struggling with depression or another mental illness. It is important for you and your child with diabetes to understand how drugs or alcohol can impact blood glucose values and how they can interfere with your teen's ability to manage his or her diabetes. Your teen's diabetes healthcare team should educate your child about the impact of drugs and alcohol on diabetes and review how your teen can stay safe. If your teen seems to have a problem with drugs or alcohol abuse/dependence, it is important that you find a counselor that can work with your teen.

Depression

It is not uncommon for individuals with diabetes, or any chronic condition, to experience depression. Several research studies have found that individuals with diabetes are at a 2 times higher risk of experiencing depression than individuals without diabetes. Hood and colleagues studied 145 youths with type 1 diabetes and found that 15% of them scored above the cutoff for clinical symptoms of depression, which is about 2 times higher than children without diabetes.

Some of the common symptoms of depression include:

- A pervasive depressed or saddened mood or irritability
- Lack of interest in activities that used to provide pleasure
- Sleep problems (sleeping too much or too little)

- Appetite changes (hungry all the time or not hungry at all)
- Weight changes
- Changes in academic performance or signs that the child/teen no longer wants to participate in sports or other activities
- Less motivation to manage diabetes

It is important to point out that some of the symptoms of high blood glucose values, like mood changes and irritability, resemble some of the symptoms of depression, so if you are worried about your child's mood, you may want to check his or her blood glucose.

If you are worried that your child may be depressed, it is important to talk to your child's pediatrician and/or diabetes healthcare team. Your child's diabetes healthcare team should be able to make a referral to a mental health counselor who can make a proper assessment. It is also important for a trained professional to assess whether you child is having any harmful or suicidal thoughts. When an individual is depressed, he or she may engage in self mutilating behaviors and have thoughts about death. If you are worried that your child is suicidal, you should take your child to the nearest emergency room or call 911 for an emergency evaluation. It is essential to note that suicidal children with diabetes should not be in charge of their own insulin administration for safety reasons.

There are several treatments for depression. One common method to treat depression is mental health counseling that involves an approach called cognitive behavioral therapy, or CBT. CBT is an approach that examines a person's thinking patterns to help the patient redirect negative thinking patterns into more positive thinking patterns, because it is believed that a person's thinking patterns influences one's behavior. Another part of CBT involves making behavioral strategies based on the patient's treatment goals. One of the main goals of therapy for individuals with depression is to feel more in control of their lives. Some individuals also benefit from taking medication, such as an antidepressant. If you think your child may need medication to help treat his or her depression, schedule an appointment with a child psychiatrist who is trained in this area. If your child is prescribed an antidepressant medication, you will want to monitor whether the antidepressant affects your child's appetite, because this could affect his or her diabetes. You should note that if your child is depressed, he or she will probably benefit from additional support and help from you for diabetes management tasks.

Anxiety

Some children and teens with diabetes experience symptoms of anxiety. One study by Grigsby and colleagues looked at several studies that examined the prevalence of anxiety in adults with diabetes. Grigsby and colleagues found that 14% of patients, or 1 in 7 adults with diabetes, met the criteria for generalized anxiety disorder. Some common symptoms of anxiety include:

- Frequent worrying
- Restlessness
- Fatigue
- Difficulty concentrating
- Irritability
- Sleep problems

Some diabetes-specific anxieties may include a fear of low blood glucose values or high blood glucose values. Some other diabetes-specific anxieties include a fear of insulin injections, pump site changes, or finger-sticks. Some individuals also worry about long-term health outcomes, healthcare provider visits, or getting blood work done in the lab. If you think your child or teen is experiencing either non-diabetes-specific anxieties or diabetes-specific anxieties, you need to address this with your child's diabetes healthcare team. The team can make a referral to a mental health specialist who can decide if your child needs follow-up treatment. The effective treatments for anxiety are similar to the treatments mentioned earlier for depression, which include mental health counseling, and may involve the use of antidepressant or antianxiety medication. Additionally, it is vital to note that some individuals who experience anxiety say that their anxiety symptoms are similar to the symptoms they feel when they are having a low blood glucose. This is why one should check a blood glucose when feeling particularly anxious, as they may be experiencing hypoglycemia.

Eating Disorders and Disordered Eating

Another challenge that some families face is when their child displays disordered eating behavior or is diagnosed with an eating disorder. *Disordered eating* would be classified as a less severe eating disturbance that does not meet the criteria for anorexia nervosa or bulimia nervosa. An *eating disorder* is a severe eating disturbance that meets the criteria for anorexia nervosa or bulimia nervosa. Disordered eating behaviors can range in severity and seem to be a risk factor for an eating disorder. Therefore, early diagnosis and treatment of disordered eating behavior may help reduce risk of an eating disorder.

In one study, Colton and colleagues studied 106 girls with type 1 diabetes who were between the ages of 9-13. They found that at the beginning of the study 14% of youth endorsed disordered eating behavior. The authors in this study defined disordered eating as:

- Dieting to control weight
- Binge eating
- Purging
- Presence of an eating disorder

Disordered eating and eating disorders can be very dangerous. In the context of diabetes, disordered eating and eating disorders can lead to suboptimal diabetes control, which can then lead to negative long-term health outcomes. Some individuals with diabetes restrict their insulin use to lose weight. If your child or teen is omitting insulin for weight loss, it is extremely dangerous. Goebel-Fabbri and colleagues found that when women engaged in insulin omission for weight loss, they experienced an increased risk of diabetes complications, shortened life span and mortality. If you suspect that your child or teen is struggling with disordered eating or may have an eating disorder, talk to your child's healthcare team and ask for a referral to a mental health counselor that specializes in eating disorders so your child can receive counseling if deemed necessary.

Summary

Managing diabetes is not easy, so you and your child may face certain challenges and pitfalls along the way. Remember that it is important to ask your child's diabetes healthcare team for help, and pursue mental health counseling when necessary. There are several strategies and treatments available to help you and your child with whatever diabetes challenges and obstacles that you may experience along the way.

References and Resources

Colton PA, Olmsted MP, Daneman AC, Rydall AC, Rodin GM. Natural history and predictors of disturbed eating behaviour in girls with type 1 diabetes. *Diabetic Medicine*. 2007; 24:424-429.

Hood KH, Huestis S, Maher A, Butler D, Volkening L, Laffel, LMB. Depressive symptoms in children and adolescents with type 1 diabetes. *Diabetes Care*. 2006;29(6):1389-1391.

Goebel-Fabbri AE, Fikkan J, Franko DL, Pearson K, Anderson BJ, Weinger K. Insulin restriction and associated morbidity and mortality in women with type 1 diabetes. *Diabetes Care*. 2008;31:415-419.

Grigsby AB, Anderson RJ, Freedland KE, Clouse RE, Lustman PJ. Prevalence of anxiety in adults with diabetes: a systematic review. *J Psychosom Res*. 2002;53(6):1053-1060.

Web sites:

- The Joslin Diabetes Center: www.joslin.org
  - Joslin Diabetes Center Discussion Boards: http://forums.joslin.org/

- Children with Diabetes.com: www.childrenwithdiabetes.com
- American Diabetes Association (ADA): www.diabetes.org
  - ADA online community for children and teens: tracker.diabetes.org
- Juvenile Diabetes Research Foundation (JDRF) International: www.jdrf.org
  - Online diabetes community created by JDRF: juvenation.org

15

School, Camp, Travel, and Other Special Events

Kids with diabetes go to school, parties, sleepovers, camp, as well as get their drivers licenses, and travel near and far. Depending on how long your child has had diabetes or how old he or she is, your comfort level when you are separated from him or her may vary. School, parties, camp, grandma's and grandpa's house, vacation, and learning to drive all make up life's adventures for your child. Having diabetes should not prevent him or her from full participation in these events of childhood; it just takes more planning to help ensure that these experiences go smoothly. You will need to help others learn how to take care of your child's diabetes management so that life can be "normal." In this chapter you will find information, tips, and strategies for these special events and circumstances.

School

School is a big part of your child's life. Though a small number of kids are home-schooled, most children still go off in the morning to spend their day with friends, classmates, teachers, school nurses, school bus drivers, and cafeteria workers. Though diabetes management in the school environment can present challenges to both your family and school personnel, they are challenges that can be met and resolved with great success. Teachers, school nurses, and other school personnel are key partners in your child's success in learning and growing. They need to have an understanding of current diabetes management plans, the individual nature of care, and how diabetes affects the whole child. Establishing a relationship with school personnel will allow you to work as a team to create the unique plan that is required to ensure that your child is safe at school.

Preparation, education, and open communication are key factors in creating a positive, safe and enriching school environment for your child. With the goal being to create a safe, healthy and happy learning environment for your child, you want your school's staff to be knowledgeable and aware of your child's medical needs. It is also important to become knowledgeable about your child's rights in the school and what the school's legal responsibilities are with regard to diabetes management. Several web sites are listed in the References and Resources section at the end of this chapter that provide useful information regarding your child's rights and the schools' responsibilities.

Federal Laws Addressing Diabetes in the School Setting

To be proactive, be informed about your child's rights in school. There are 3 federal laws that protect students with diabetes in the school setting. They provide a framework to address your child's medical management during the school day and during extracurricular school activities. The following is a summary of each of these laws.

- *Section 504 of the Rehabilitation Act of 1973 (Section 504)*
  - The 504 Plan sets out an agreement for making sure the student has the same access to education as do other children. It is a tool that can be used to ensure that the student, the parents/guardians, and school personnel understand their responsibilities and to work out potential problems or misunderstandings ahead of time. A 504 Plan may be developed as a result of a request by the school, the parents'/guardians' request or in response to a problem with the student's care at school.
    - The 504 Plan is a legally binding document.
    - Useful Website: ndep.nih.gov/diabetes/pubs/youth_NDEPSchoolGuide.pdf
- *Individuals with Disabilities Education Act (IDEA)*
  - Some children with diabetes may be served under the Individuals with Disabilities in Education Act, also known as IDEA. To qualify under IDEA, the student's academic performance must be directly affected by a disability to the

point that the student requires special education and related services. If your child qualifies under this Act, the school plan developed would be an Individualized Education Program or IEP. Typically, an IEP is more specific than a 504 Plan with regard to the student's academic needs. The IEP should be developed by the parent/guardian, the child's diabetes healthcare team and school personnel.

    - The IEP is a legally binding document.
    - Useful Website: idea.ed.gov

- *The Americans with Disabilities Act (ADA)*
  - This law expressly prohibits all schools from discriminating against people with disabilities.
    - Useful Website: www.ada.gov

An annual meeting with the principal, school nurse, and teacher(s) provides an opportunity to update school personnel on new information regarding your child's diabetes as well as ensuring that new teachers are up to speed about how to handle diabetes-specific situations in the school. This type of meeting is also necessary when your child is newly diagnosed with diabetes, or if aspects of his or her diabetes management change. Additionally, developing a written plan will provide concrete guidance for school personnel that they can continue to refer to as needed throughout the year. Such a plan also allows information to be provided to many different school personnel, thus ensuring that all who care for your child are well informed. The American Diabetes Association recommends 2 elements to this plan:

- *Information Packet*
  - Written information about diabetes that the school personnel may find helpful (*e.g.* flyers, brochures, reference lists, articles, or useful web sites).
- *Diabetes Care/HealthCare Plan*
  - A written outline of your child's diabetes treatment plan. This can potentially take the form of a Diabetes Medical Management Plan (DMMP) which can be developed into a 504 plan or IDEA/IEP plan

Table 15-1. Written Diabetes Care Plans

DMMP	504 Plan	IDEA
The Diabetes Medical Management Plan (DMMP) specifies your child's diabetes needs throughout the day. This should be reviewed and updated each school year or upon a change in your child's diabetes regimen, a change in school circumstances (*e.g.*, a change in schedule), or at the request of the student, parents/guardians or teacher. For more information on DMMPs go to: www.ndep.nih.gov/diabetes/pubs/Youth_NDEPSchoolGuide.pdf	A *504 Plan* is the term used for a plan developed under Section 504 of the Rehabilitation Act of 1973. Information from the DMMP can be used as the foundation for developing a 504 Plan. One of the major differences between a DMMP and a 504 Plan is that a 504 Plan is a legally binding document. The 504 Plan sets out an agreement for making sure your child has the same access to education as do other children. It defines responsibilities of all parties. A 504 Plan may be developed as a result of a request by the school, the parents/guardians or in response to a problem with the student's care at school. For more information on 504s go to: www.dol.gov/oasam/regs/statutes/sec504.htm or www.diabetes.org/advocacy-andlegalresources/discrimination/school/504plan.jsp	To qualify under IDEA, the student's academic performance must be directly affected by a disability to the point that the student requires special education and related services. Each child's IEP must include the supplementary aids and services to be provided for the child, a statement of the program modifications or supports for school personnel that will be provided for the child, and how progress will be measured over time. If your child has an IEP then he or she does not need a 504 Plan. All necessary information will be written into the IEP. For more information go to: www.ed.gov/parents/needs/speced/iepguide or www.ideapractices.org

A more detailed description of the above is available in the book *Helping the Student with Diabetes Succeed – A Guide for School Personnel*, available from the National Diabetes Education Program online at: www.ndep.nih.gov/diabetes/pubs/Youth_NDEPSchoolGuide.pdf

The 3 types of written plans are described in more detail in Table 15-1.

Classroom Presentations

Depending on your child's age and temperament, he or she may be interested in a classroom presentation about diabetes so that the other students can learn about it. Some children are more private about their diabetes than other children, so they may or may not be comfortable with the idea of a classroom presentation about diabetes. Make sure that you discuss the details of the presentation with your child and your child's teacher, and discuss who will be doing the presentation. The presentation should be brief and age appropriate. Depending on the age of your child, it may be easier to read a children's book about diabetes, such as *Taking Diabetes to School* by Kim Gosselin, instead of giving a more formal presentation. Education such as this can prevent some of the potential teasing and questions that the other students may ask your child throughout the school year.

Field Trips

Field trips can provide great learning opportunities, but they can sometimes present challenges for families living with diabetes. Children with diabetes should participate in all school activities, including field trips. Unfortunately, staffing and budget issues may mean that a school nurse is not available to go on the trip. If your child attends public school and the nurse will not be on the trip, the school must arrange for a trained staff member to be available for your child's diabetes care. Private schools, however, are not always required to provide this accommodation, so a parent or other caregiver may need to go on the field trip. As soon as you are notified of an upcoming field trip, contact the school to discuss whether the school nurse or another staff member will be traveling with the school group or if you will be expected to attend. If you will not be accompanying your child's class, make sure that an adult knows about the specifics of your child's diabetes management. Even if your child is able to monitor blood glucose and administer insulin on his or her own, a knowledgeable adult should be available to supervise these tasks. The excitement and novelty of a school trip may distract your child and diabetes tasks could be forgotten. It will need to be determined who will carry your child's diabetes supplies during the trip. Staff and chaperones supervising the trip should be familiar with symptoms of hypoglycemia and hyperglycemia and what action to take should those symptoms arise. In addition, staff will need to have contact information so that they will know who to reach and how, in the event of questions or emergencies.

It is important to pack all the necessary supplies that your child may need. Make sure that your child has a kit made up of the following:

- Blood glucose meter and
  - strips
  - lancing device
  - lancets
- Alcohol swabs (for use if hand-washing facilities will not be available)

- Sharps container (sharps containers are available at many pharmacies but an empty film canister or plastic drink bottle also works well)
- Food
  - fast-acting carbohydrates
  - snacks
- Glucagon
- Insulin and a means to administer it
- Medical identification worn by your child

Insulin and syringes or insulin pen and needles should also be packed. Even if your child will not be scheduled for an insulin dose during the trip, situations like a high blood glucose, a broken insulin pump, or an unexpected delay in the trip return can make an insulin shot necessary.

In the event that your child's pump or injection site is not working, make sure that there is insulin, a delivery device other than the pump, and ketone strips as well as someone to help with an insulin injection. Another possibility is to pack an additional infusion set in case the pump site needs to be changed. However, this may complicate the issue; if so, just plan on your child getting his or her insulin from a syringe or pen. If your child's diabetes care includes a basal/bolus insulin plan or an insulin pump, ensure that a trained adult will be helping to count carbohydrates for meals and snacks.

If you are packing lunch, snacks, or dinner for your child, you can make carbohydrate counting easier for the staff by writing the carbohydrate counts on the packaging of each food item. In situations where food will be provided by the school or at the field trip location, it may be helpful to call ahead and determine the carbohydrate content of the food that will be served or send a carbohydrate counting book with the staff. The age of your child will come into play as to how much assistance he needs.

School field trips require families to do extra planning. Although the packing list above may feel long, once you have gathered the items for one or two trips, you'll feel comfortable doing so and it will no longer feel overwhelming. Taking the time to prepare before the trip will enable the school to properly manage your child's diabetes so that he or she can enjoy the unique learning experiences.

Academic and Standardized Testing

Many schools take part in standardized testing. Plan ahead of time whether your child may need any particular accommodations to the school's testing procedures. In your child's school plan, you can specify any particular needs your child may have. For example, you may want your child to be allowed additional time to check and treat blood glucose levels and to use the bathroom or water fountain when necessary. If your child will be doing the testing outside of his or her school, you may want to contact the academic testing site to see if there is a particular form that you are required to fill out to have these accommodations in place. Often this is an issue that will be taken up directly through the testing center rather than the school. For information on SAT type exams, the College Board provides information on its web site at: professionals.collegeboard.com/testing/sat-reasoning/register/accomodations.

Holidays and Parties

Holiday celebrations and parties are an important part of most peoples' lives. These special occasions typically include foods and activities that require planning for optimal diabetes management. Remember that children with diabetes do not have to give up birthday parties and holiday gatherings to keep blood glucose levels in control. As with many other aspects of diabetes management, planning, communication, and preparation are the keys to balancing special events and diabetes needs.

When your child is invited to a party or special event, find out as much as you can about the foods and activities planned for the event. What kinds of food will be served and at what time? Will the children be active at the party, playing sports or games, or will they be quieter, watching a movie or doing arts and crafts? If the party will take place away from home or at school, speaking to the host or teacher in advance will help you to determine how to balance the food, activities and insulin. Depending on the situation, you may need to adjust your child's insulin dose or pack a snack. Communication is particularly important if you will not be attending the party, since you will need to make sure that someone is able to look out for and help your child.

Planning is everything. First consider what your child's activity level will be. For example, if your child is attending a pool party and will be swimming a lot, he or she may actually need the carbohydrates in the cake or cookies to prevent hypoglycemia. For less active celebrations, you may need to plan to give your child more insulin to cover the foods he or she eats. The timing of the party and when food will be served is also important to think about. Holiday meals, in particular, tend to be served at unusual times, such as mid-afternoon. You may need to temporarily change your child's insulin plan for that day. If you are not confident in making such adjustments on your own, contact your diabetes healthcare team for advice in advance of the day.

Blood glucose monitoring is especially important during parties and holiday gatherings, since special foods, time changes in meals, excitement, and varying physical activity levels can make blood glucose levels more difficult to predict. By having a blood glucose meter at the party and checking blood glucose before giving insulin or treating a suspected low blood glucose, it will be easier to maintain glucose control. Your child will also need access to fast-acting carbohydrates during the party, in case of low blood glucose, and you should discuss hypoglycemia and your child's usual symptoms with the party's hosts. Since party foods and exercise can have prolonged effects on blood glucose, you should monitor more frequently for a few hours after the celebration.

Halloween

Halloween is one of the most cherished holidays of childhood. Using a few simple strategies may help you and your child enjoy Halloween activities without sacrificing reasonable diabetes management. For example, you may want to talk to your child's healthcare team about how to cover certain treats with insulin. While trick-or-treating, let your child eat some candy. She is getting a lot of exercise by walking, climbing stairs, etc. Your child will be much less likely to snack on large amounts of candy if it is kept out of sight. Some families also choose to plan an exchange program for Halloween candy. For instance, you can have your child trade his extra candy for a new stuffed animal or a special family outing. This sort of strategy works best if you involve all the children in the family, so that the child with diabetes does not feel singled out. As with many of the situations discussed in this chapter, planning and preparation can make Halloween go much more smoothly and be a positive experience for your child.

Family and Friends

Remember when you were a new parent? Remember when you needed the support of family and friends? Now that your child has diabetes, the need for caregiving support has only grown. Given the extra effort needed to take care of a child with diabetes, the support of relatives, loved ones, family friends, and trusted babysitters can be extremely beneficial for you and your family. All caregivers need a break from time to time, and with proper planning and organization you should be able to leave your child in the care of trusted individuals. Family members, neighbors, or babysitters that took care of your child before he or she was diagnosed with diabetes are often willing to learn to take on certain diabetes tasks and care for your child. If you do not already have friends or family who are willing and able to learn how to manage your child's diabetes, you may be able to find caregivers in your community. Networking with other parents of children with diabetes may allow you to exchange childcare from time to time, or they may be able to introduce you to babysitters already familiar with diabetes care because they have diabetes or may have a sibling with diabetes. It may also be helpful to contact a local nursing school to connect with students who are familiar with giving medications and injections and interested in babysitting.

Once you have identified the people who will be helping to care for your child, they need to be educated on the basics of diabetes and the specifics of your child's diabetes treatment plan. Those with a medical background or who are familiar with diabetes may be able to become familiar with your child's diabetes care regimen in a relatively short amount of time, but caregivers who are less experienced with diabetes may need more training.

Some hospitals and diabetes centers offer programs to help relatives and babysitters learn how to care for diabetes, but many families choose to train caregivers themselves. If you are anxious about leaving your child in someone else's care, start small; teach a trusted person to recognize and treat low blood glucose and try going out for an hour or two. Once you and the caregiver are comfortable while you are away for a short time, you may feel more comfortable leaving for longer stretches.

Whether you will be away from your child for an hour or a weekend, be sure your child's caregiver has all the information and supplies to care for your child, including information about blood glucose monitoring, meal planning, insulin administration, and treatment of low and high blood glucose. Just like you used to do before your child had diabetes, provide emergency phone numbers and anything else that you think is necessary for the caregiver to know. Some parents ask that the caregiver call before giving insulin or to discuss their child's blood glucose. You may also want to ask the caregiver to write down any insulin that is given, along with any blood glucose readings and what time they occurred.

Having a support network of people who are capable of caring for your child will allow you to take a break from the demands of diabetes, and allow you that same sense of freedom you experienced when you were first able to leave your child in the hands of a trusted caregiver. Know that with some education regarding diabetes management, many of these trusted sources can still take good care of your child. Having such a support network will help make living with diabetes in your family much easier and will be safer for your child.

Travel

Traveling can present challenges in the best of circumstances. Add diabetes into the mix and you know that planning and preparation for diabetes care are important for a successful trip. Think carefully about what supplies your child will need and in what quantities, where supplies will be kept, who will carry them, and who will be responsible for all the parts of your child's diabetes regimen.

As you begin to prepare for a trip, use the following questions to help plan for your child's travel.

- How long will the trip last?
- Who will be responsible for my child's diabetes care? (*e.g.*, parent, nurse, teacher, etc.)

- What food, if any will be part of the trip?
- When will blood glucose monitoring be performed and by whom?
- What diabetes supplies will be needed for the trip?
- Who will be responsible for carrying and keeping track of diabetes supplies?
- How will the planned activities of the trip (*e.g.*, food, exercise, time zone changes, long transportation time, etc.) affect the insulin doses my child will need before, during, or after the trip?
- What kind of medical identification will my child wear?

In addition to these questions, consider contacting your child's diabetes healthcare team to discuss questions or concerns in advance so that you can avoid potential problems. Use the travel checklist at the end of this section to help you prepare.

The following sections describe a few specific kinds of trips that your child may make and the special considerations that need to be made.

Sports Trips

Most sports trips do not include a school nurse and there may be many you are not attending yourself. Given this, your child's Diabetes Plan should include details for:

- Training of coaches, etc.
- Signs and treatments for low blood glucose
- A plan in the event of a severe low blood glucose
- Frequent blood glucose monitoring appropriate for the trip

Sleepovers and Overnight Trips

Sleepovers where you are not attending are a part of childhood. For sleepovers close to home, you may choose to go to the friend's house when your child needs insulin. For trips that are farther away, you will need to put together a plan for insulin administration, meal planning, and blood glucose monitoring. It is advantageous to have an adult to supervise insulin doses, along with ensuring your child's blood glucose gets checked. Cell phones and computers are wonderful tools for other parents to get in touch with you to do things like determining the insulin dose, to answering questions and giving some long-distance diabetes education.

In situations where your child will be traveling without you, remember to determine who will be responsible for helping your child with his or her diabetes management. A version of the Diabetes Care plan may be helpful. Add the diabetes tasks to any other special notes that you send along with your child.

Vacations and Family Trips

Preparing for a family trip or vacation always takes a lot of planning and forethought. Having everything needed to manage your child's diabetes while you are away from home will help to make the trip go smoothly. Plan if you will be:

- Traveling to a different time zone
- Traveling to an area with extreme high or low temperatures
- Very active or not active at all (a hiking trip or a trip to visit an elderly relative)
- Flying
- Unaware of where medical and pharmacy services are available
- Traveling abroad (learn how to say your child has diabetes or needs juice in the language of the country in which you'll be traveling)

Due to airport security regulations about liquids, you may not be able to carry juice boxes or glucose gel through screening checkpoints, so be sure to have items like glucose tablets or jelly beans. Checking blood glucose often will help you to know how all the variables of travel are affecting your child and what changes to his or her treatment plan may need to be made.

Table 15-2 lists diabetes supplies that are needed for travel. It is a resource you can adapt to the specific needs of your child's trip.

Table 15-2. Travel Checklist of Diabetes Supplies

NOTE: You may not need every item on this list for every trip. These are guidelines that can be adapted for your specific situation.

Remember to keep all diabetes supplies with you. ***Do not*** pack them in your checked luggage.

Prescription items should have original pharmacy labels.

☐ Blood Glucose Meter(s)	**Pump Supplies:**
☐ Batteries for the Meter	☐ Infusion Sets
☐ Strips for the Meter	☐ Reservoirs
☐ Urine Ketone Strips or Blood Ketone Strips and Meter	☐ Inserter
☐ Lancets	☐ IV Prep Pads
☐ Lancet Device	☐ Extra Battery
☐ Alcohol Wipes	☐ Pump company contact information in case of pump problems
☐ Log Book/Sheets	
☐ Insulin (extra vials/cartridges of each type used)	
☐ Syringes/Pens and Needle Tips	
☐ Glucagon Emergency Kit with Syringe	
☐ Treatment for Low Blood Glucose	
☐ Snacks	
☐ Medical Alert Bracelet or Necklace	
☐ Emergency Telephone Numbers	
☐ Travel Letter	
☐ Emergency contact numbers, including how to contact your child's healthcare team	

Driving? Of Course!

Getting a driver's license is one of the many transitions to adulthood. The freedom and flexibility of driving brings responsibilities. People with diabetes can most certainly get their driver's license. However, because people who take insulin are at risk for low blood glucose levels, teens with diabetes often need a letter addressed to their state's Department of Motor Vehicles, from their healthcare team, stating that their diabetes will not pose a problem for driving safely.

Before your child drives, make sure you review the "rules of the road" below:

1. Be sure you are wearing your medical identification.
2. Make sure that you check your blood glucose whether you will be driving for a short or long excursion.
    a. Determine with your healthcare team the blood glucose level that is "out-of-range" for driving and do not drive if your blood glucose is in that range.
    b. No matter where you are going – if you have a low blood glucose – wait until you have treated that low and are in a safe blood glucose level range before driving.
    c. Always keep fast-acting carbohydrate (such as glucose tablets, juice, lifesavers) as well as snacks in the car. Know which carbohydrates will "survive" the high and low temperatures of the seasons.

How often should you check your blood glucose while driving? Carry enough diabetes supplies with you to be able to check your blood glucose at least every 2 hours. If you are driving and feel low, pull safely into a parking space on the street or parking area. If it is not possible to immediately pull to the side of the road, start treating the symptoms of a "low" without waiting to check a blood glucose. It is better to err on the side of safety.

Supplies to keep in the car include:

1. Blood glucose meter, lancets, strips (make sure that the inside of the car will not be out of the temperature range for the meter and strips).
2. Fast acting carbohydrate such as glucose tablets, juice, etc.
3. Snacks such as granola bars, crackers, etc.

Some web sites you may want to check out:

- American Diabetes Association - State Regulation of Drivers with Diabetes: http://www.diabetes.org/advocacy-and-legalresources/discrimination/drivers/pvt-licensemap.jsp
- US Department of Transportation Website: http://www.nhtsa.dot.gov/people/injury/olddrive/Diabetes%20Web/
- dLife: http://www.dlife.com/dLife/do/ShowContent/daily_living/traveling_with_diabetes/driving.html

Driving is a huge responsibility — protect yourself and others by driving safely, paying attention to the laws of driving, speed limits, pedestrians, and your diabetes management.

Camp

There aren't many experiences quite like summer camp. Camp is a place where children are given new opportunities to learn, have fun and meet many new friends. It is a unique environment for children and a time they will always remember. Living with diabetes brings forth a new set of concerns and reservations that families may not have thought about before their child was diagnosed. In this section, you will read about both diabetes and regular camps — both day and sleepover camps. Each offers a different opportunity. Which is right for your family and your child?

Diabetes Camp

In 1925, four years after Drs. Banting and Best discovered insulin, the first diabetes camp opened. Having diabetes means your child has different needs and responsibilities than other children who do not have diabetes. For children and adolescents with diabetes, 50–51 weeks a year are spent in the "real world," where diabetes self-management tasks are not the norm among their peers. For one or two weeks a year, diabetes camp provides a rare opportunity of being the norm, and sharing experiences with others who live with and understand diabetes.

As with all summer camps, children at diabetes camp enjoy many activities, from canoeing to wilderness hikes to talent shows. What sets diabetes camps apart from other camps is that the counselors, staff, and medical teams are specifically trained to take care of children with diabetes. Frequently, many of the counselors have diabetes themselves. Medical teams anticipate the daily diabetes management tasks that are required, including multiple blood glucose checks throughout the day and designated times to administer insulin. The staff provides an environment where your child will be safe so that he or she can focus on having fun. Campers benefit from: meeting other children and staff with diabetes, learning about new ways to manage diabetes, and being

Table 15-3. Review of a Diabetes Camp's Services
• Staff and counselors with diabetes knowledge and understanding
• On site medical team including doctor and nurse available
• Medical facilities and supplies
• Nutrition information and guidance for individual meal plans
• Close monitoring of blood glucose and established schedules for blood glucose checks
• Administration of insulin including insulin by injection and by insulin pump
• Knowledge of varying insulin regimens and pump therapy/maintenance
• Overall focus on safety
• Emergency procedure plans
• Activities that have built-in accommodations for children with diabetes
Adapted from: American Diabetes Association. *Getting the Most Out of Diabetes Camps: A Guide for Parents and Kids.* Alexandria, VA: American Diabetes Association; 2002.

exposed to new tools and therapies. Healthcare professionals gain diabetes research and clinical experience by participating in camps. Campers' parents receive a welcome vacation from the daily tasks of diabetes management.

Diabetes camp can also provide an educational experience for many children. This process of learning is usually very natural at diabetes camp. It may happen on the way to lunch when it is time to check blood glucose or at story time in the cabin just before bed when one of the campers is having a low blood glucose. Most diabetes camp programs offer 5-day to 2-week sessions. For further information on diabetes camps visit specific diabetes camps or the following web sites:

- American Diabetes Associations Websites: www.diabetescamps.org
- Diabetes Education & Camping Association: www.diabetescamps.org
- Children With Diabetes: www.childrenwithdiabetes.com

A concern that many families have about diabetes camp is whether the staff is qualified to manage their child's diabetes. As you research camps in your area, Table 15-3 provides some suggestions of topics to discuss to ensure you are comfortable with the facility.

In addition, there are diabetes camps that are day camps and some that are overnight camps, so this is something to keep in mind when you are planning the best camp for your child.

Day Camp

A day camp is a program run during the day for children typically between the ages of 4-12 years old. You may find countless types of activities your child can partake in at day camp, and often these programs run anywhere from one to eight weeks in length. Day camp is a great chance for a younger child to begin his or her camp experience. Since everyone goes home at the end of the day, it may be less stressful for your child than overnight camp.

Sleepover Camp

Sleepover camps typically last one to four weeks, but can last for up to eight weeks. Your child will spend all day with fellow campers trying new activities and events, and end the day in a cabin with other campers and counselors. Sleepover camp is often a child's first experience away from home and this may be difficult for both you and your child. Many children feel homesick at some point during sleepover camp and this should be expected. Days are filled with various activities and evenings are usually spent participating in planned events

Day Camp vs. Sleepover Camp

Knowing whether your child is prepared for day camp or sleepover camp may be dependent upon your child's age, emotional readiness, and interests. Each child is unique and a great way for your family to decide which camp is best for your child is to talk about the options together. Ask your child what type of camp he or she is interested in and what type of experience he or she wants. If you are unsure of what camp may be like, you may want to go visit a camp close to home. Many camps love having families visit on a planned day or weekend to create excitement and show you their facilities. This can be a very positive experience for both you and your child where you can see what the camp is like and decide if it is a place where your child will be comfortable, safe, and have fun.

Preparing for Camp

Once you have decided to send your child to camp, it is time to gather all of the necessary information so that the camp staff is fully prepared to take care of your child and manage his or her diabetes. You will receive a packet of information once your child has been given a spot for a particular session. Be sure to look through the packet and see exactly what types of forms are enclosed and what the camp staff will be expecting from you.

Look for the medical form that asks for specific information about your child's health. You will need a physician's signature on this form so it is important to read the form carefully. You want to include as much information as possible. The more details you can provide the camp staff about your child, the better prepared they will be to take care of him or her. You will want to include any medical information about your child, including diabetes management information as well as additional health concerns (such as allergies, etc.). The diabetes information that you provide should include specific information on how your child manages his or her diabetes each day. Remember to include information about the number of blood glucose checks, insulin administration, treatment for hypoglycemia (preferred treatment and carbohydrate amount including glucagon administration), treatment for hyperglycemia, and meal planning information. Plan what diabetes supplies you will need to leave at your child's camp. Also, be aware that while at camp, children often experience different blood glucose values than you might expect at home. Your child's change in activity may impact how much insulin he or she needs and the frequency of blood glucose monitoring.

Before the first day of camp begins, here are some other items to consider:

- Talking with your child to be sure that he knows what to expect from camp and how to handle any questions or concerns, especially if this is his or her first camp experience. Be open about feeling homesick and discuss what your child could do if he or she feels homesick (*e.g.*, turning to a new friend or counselor, staying busy or, if going to an overnight camp, writing letters).

- Talking to the medical staff at the camp to discuss your child's diabetes management plan and needs.
- Making sure that the camp staff has all of your emergency contact information.
- In addition to packing the diabetes supplies that you know your child will need, pack extra diabetes supplies.
- Remember that if camp doesn't work out, that is okay! There is always next year and at least your child tried something new.

All of these steps will lay the groundwork for your child to have a positive and fun experience at summer camp. Camp can be a truly enriching experience for children. Although having a child with diabetes certainly adds additional challenges when planning for camp, with the proper tools and knowledge, your child can have a wonderful experience.

Summary

Planning your child's diabetes management for school, travel, and holidays takes time and energy. However, children with diabetes will benefit from being able to participate in all the activities and events that other children experience. With planning, preparation, and good communication, your child can thrive whether at school, at a sleepover or on a family vacation without sacrificing good diabetes care.

References and Resources

Gosselin, K. *Taking Diabetes to School: Special Kids in School*. New York: JayJo Books; 2004

American Diabetes Association. *Getting the Most Out of Diabetes Camps: A Guide for Parents and Kids*. Alexandria, VA: American Diabetes Association; 2002.

Helping the Student with Diabetes Succeed A Guide for School Personnel (available at http://ndep.nih.gov/materials/pubs/schoolguide.pdf)

Web sites:

- American Diabetes Association Advocacy and Legal Resources: www.diabetes.org/advocacy-and-legalresources
- American Diabetes Association School Position Statement: care.diabetesjournals.org
- American Association of Diabetes Educators Position Statement: www.diabeteseducator.org
- National Diabetes Education Program: Helping the Student with Diabetes Succeed: A *Comprehensive Guide for Families and School Personnel.*: ndep.nih.gov
- College Board: professionals.collegeboard.com
- Children With Diabetes: www.childrenwithdiabetes.com
- Juvenile Diabetes Research Foundation: www.jdrf.org
- American Diabetes Association - State Regulation of Drivers with Diabetes: www.diabetes.org
- US Department of Transportation Website: www.nhtsa.dot.gov
- dLife: www.dlife.com
- American Diabetes Associations Camp Websites at: www.diabetes camps.org/
- Diabetes Education & Camping Association at www.diabetescamps.org/
- Children With Diabetes Camp Information: www.childrenwithdiabetes.com

16

Long-Term Complications and Co-Morbidities

Individuals with diabetes mellitus are at risk for a number of long-term complications. The long-term complications of diabetes are generally classified into one of two categories: microvascular, which involve small blood vessels, or macrovascular, which involve large blood vessels.

Microvascular Complications

The microvascular complications of diabetes include damage to the back of the eyes (*i.e.*, retina), the kidneys, and peripheral nerves. These complications are called diabetic retinopathy, nephropathy, and neuropathy, respectively. These complications develop gradually over years. The encouraging news, however, is that an important study called the Diabetes Control and Complications Trial (DCCT) clearly demonstrated that optimal blood glucose control reduces the risk for microvascular complications by as much as 50 percent. This is one of the many reasons that your child's diabetes healthcare team works hard with you to help regulate your child's blood glucose levels.

There are routine screening lab tests to detect complications at an early stage when treatment can stop, slow down, or reverse the disease processes. Most of the screening recommendations outlined in the rest of this chapter pertain specifically to children with type 1 diabetes. If your child has type 2 diabetes, his or her medical provider will likely recommend performing a number of these screening tests shortly after diagnosis.

Tables 16-1, 16-2 and 16-3 summarize the background, risk factors, screening recommendations, and treatments for the various microvascular complications.

Table 16-1. Retinopathy: Background, Screening, and Treatment

Background	Risk Factors	Screening Recommendations	Treatment
Diabetes-associated retinopathy is a disorder that affects the small blood vessels that supply blood to the back of the eye. This complication is categorized into stages based on the degree of severity. Fortunately, vigilant screening allows detection of retinopathy at early stages, most often allowing treatment before vision is affected.	Poor blood glucose control, high blood pressure, elevated protein in the urine, elevated lipid levels, smoking, longer duration of diabetes, and pregnancy are all known risk factors for retinopathy.	Your child's medical provider will likely recommend that an eye care professional skilled in the care of children and adolescents with diabetes examine your child. The first eye examination should usually be obtained once your child is $\geq$ 10 years of age and has had diabetes for 3-5 years. For children diagnosed as infants or toddlers, often the young child may have a first eye exam upon entering grade school. These eye exams require that drops be placed into the eyes to allow for a full dilated eye exam. After the initial eye examination, annual routine follow-up is generally recommended. Less frequent examinations may be acceptable on the advice of an eye care professional. Any young woman with diabetes who is planning pregnancy should have an eye examination before becoming pregnant.	Lowering elevated blood pressure levels, improving poor blood glucose control, and stopping smoking all help to slow down and potentially reverse retinopathy. Laser therapy is very effective at preserving vision when a more advanced stage of sight-threatening retinopathy is present.

Table 16-2. Nephropathy: Background, Screening, and Treatment

Background	Risk Factors	Screening Recommendations	Treatment
Diabetes-associated nephropathy is a disorder that affects the small blood vessels that supply blood to the kidney. Similar to retinopathy, nephropathy is categorized into stages based on the degree of severity. A condition called microalbuminuria, which involves the release of small amounts of protein into the urine, is the earliest stage of nephropathy.	Risk factors for nephropathy include poor blood glucose control, elevated blood pressure, smoking, parental history of elevated blood pressure, and a family history of cardiovascular disease.	Your child's medical provider will likely recommend screening for nephropathy once your child is 10 years of age and/or has had diabetes for 5 years. Screening for nephropathy can be performed in a number of different ways. For example, your child's medical provider might request that your child provide a random spot urine sample during a scheduled medical visit. Alternatively, the provider may suggest performing a 24-hour urine collection for analysis or collecting a first morning urine sample. Exercise, smoking, and menstruation can all affect the results of the urine screen. In addition, your child's urinary protein excretion can vary from day to day. Therefore, if your child has an abnormal urine screen, his healthcare provider will likely recommend that the abnormal test be repeated. Even an illness or a significant low blood glucose reaction may lead to a temporary increase in urine protein.	If your child has a persistently elevated microalbumin level in his or her urine, your child's medical provider will likely recommend starting your child on a medication called an ACE inhibitor. The purpose of the medication is to try to return the level of protein in the urine to normal (if possible). If your child has microalbuminuria, it is also very important that his or her blood glucose levels be tightly regulated. Avoiding or stopping smoking, controlling blood pressure, and lowering elevated blood lipid levels (if present) are also very important ways of keeping your child's kidneys healthy. If your child's medical provider has taken all of the above steps and your child's urine screen remains abnormal, it might be recommended that a doctor who specializes in the care of the kidney see and evaluate your child.

Table 16-3. Neuropathy: Background, Screening, and Treatment

Neurologic complications of diabetes are seldom seen in the pediatric and adolescent population. Your child's healthcare provider will perform foot exams each year. Your provider may check reflexes or vibration sensation. These exams help assess a condition called peripheral neuropathy. As your child gets older, the foot exam may include a test using a microfilament. In this test, the healthcare provider checks your child's foot sensation. Another kind of neuropathy involves the central nervous system. This complication, called automatic neuropathy, is checked by carefully measuring the heart rate and blood pressure. Both peripheral and autonomic neuropathies are uncommon in children.

Macrovascular Complications

The macrovascular complications of diabetes include cardiovascular disease (CVD), cerebrovascular disease, and peripheral vascular disease. These 3 diseases involve the large blood vessels that supply the heart, brain, and periphery (*e.g.*, lower legs), respectively.

CVD is the leading cause of death and morbidity in the United States. Studies have shown that CVD begins early in life and is progressive throughout the life span. The strongest known risk factors for CVD include elevated blood pressure, high LDL (*i.e.*, bad) cholesterol, low HDL (*i.e.*, good) cholesterol, cigarette smoking, obesity, and diabetes.

Table 16-4. Hypertension (i.e., high blood pressure): Background, Screening, and Treatment

Background	Risk Factors	Screening Recommendations	Treatment
Hypertension is a risk factor for the development of many diabetes-related complications.	Studies have shown that elevated blood pressure in a parent is a major risk factor for elevated blood pressure in a child. Additional risk factors include a sedentary lifestyle, smoking, and being overweight.	At each visit, your child's blood pressure will likely be measured and reviewed by your child's medical provider. In addition, your child's medical provider is likely to ask you questions about whether or not there is a family history of elevated blood pressure. If your child is found to have elevated blood pressure, his or her medical provider will likely recommend obtaining additional laboratory tests including one for kidney function.	Treatment of elevated blood pressure is very important to keep your child healthy. If your child has elevated blood pressure, his or her medical provider will likely recommend a number of lifestyle changes. For example, it will likely be recommended that your child be placed on a meal plan consisting of no added salt. In addition, if your child is not very physically active or if your child smokes, it will likely be recommended that your child exercise more frequently and stop smoking. If your child is overweight, weight loss will likely be recommended. If your child's blood pressure target is not reached within 3-6 months, despite making the lifestyle changes outlined above, your child's medical provider will likely recommend starting a medication called an ACE inhibitor. Use of ACE inhibitors in children has been found to be safe and effective; however, they are not to be used during pregnancy.

Table 16-5. Dyslipidemia (i.e., high lipid levels): Background, Screening, and Treatment			
Background	**Risk Factors**	**Screening Recommendations**	**Treatment**
According to the National Cholesterol Education Program (NCEP) and the American Academy of Pediatrics (AAP), all children with diabetes mellitus should undergo cholesterol screening.	Family history of lipid disorders, overweight or obesity, lifestyle, unhealthy eating, and uncontrolled diabetes.	Your child's healthcare provider is likely to recommend that your child's first cholesterol screening take place after two years of age but no later than 10 years of age. A fasting lipid profile may be recommended for screening. Often lipid levels are measured at a medical visit mid-day. If the non-fasting lipid levels are abnormal, your medical provider may repeat the studies before breakfast in the fasted state. If your child's initial lipid screen is normal, it will likely be recommended that he/she be retested in 3 to 5 years.	Treatment of abnormal cholesterol levels is important to keep your child healthy. If your child has abnormal cholesterol levels, his/her medical provider will likely recommend a number of changes to your child's meal plan, including a reduction in total fat, saturated fat, and cholesterol. Lifestyle changes identical to those recommended for hypertension (*i.e.*, weight control, increased physical activity, smoking cessation, and attention to blood glucose control) are also recommended to improve lipid levels. If diet therapy and lifestyle changes are not successful, your child's medical provider might recommend starting your child on a medication to help improve his/her lipid levels.

Tables 16-4 and 16-5 summarize the background, risk factors, screening recommendations and treatments for these risk factors.

Other Long-Term Complications of Diabetes

Foot Care

Although foot problems are rare in children and adolescents with diabetes, it is valuable for your child to learn how to care for his or her feet and develop good foot care skills. It is recommended that children with type 1 diabetes have their feet examined beginning at puberty and then at least annually thereafter.

Adjustment and Psychiatric Disorders

Unfortunately, diabetes is a risk factor for adolescent psychiatric disorders, including depression and anxiety. Psychiatric illness is a serious complication of diabetes and is often associated with poor blood glucose control and recurrent hospitalization. Therefore, if you ever have concerns that your child seems anxious or depressed, it is very important that you discuss these concerns with his or her medical provider because prompt evaluation and treatment by a mental health specialist may be needed. Help is available for such conditions. Additional information regarding such disorders can be found in Chapter 14: Behavioral Pitfalls — Prevention and Early Intervention.

Eating Disorders

Eating disorders are also associated with diabetes in adolescents. Youth, especially girls, with eating disorders are more likely to have poor blood glucose control and recurrent hospitalizations. Therefore, if you ever have a suspicion that your child has an eating disorder, it is once again very important that you discuss your concerns with his or her medical provider. Additional information regarding such eating disorders and disordered eating can be found in Chapter 14: Behavioral Pitfalls — Prevention and Early Intervention.

Co-Morbidities of Diabetes

Thyroid disease

The thyroid gland is located in the neck and is responsible for the production of thyroid hormone. Thyroid hormone has many functions in the body and helps to control a person's metabolism. Increased levels of thyroid hormone tend to speed up a person's metabolism, while decreased levels of thyroid hormone tend to slow down a person's metabolism.

More than 15% of individuals with type 1 diabetes have an autoimmune thyroid disorder, which may interfere with the body's production of thyroid hormone. In fact, thyroid disease is the most common autoimmune disorder associated with type 1 diabetes. Children and adolescents with autoimmune thyroid conditions may have normal, low, or elevated levels of thyroid hormone in their blood. Children with too much thyroid hormone, a condition called hyperthyroidism, metabolize glucose differently and may have difficulty keeping their blood glucose levels steady. Children with too little thyroid hormone, a condition called hypothyroidism, might not grow well and may be predisposed to low blood glucose reactions.

If your child has type 1 diabetes, his or her medical provider might recommend screening him or her for autoimmune thyroid disease at the time of diagnosis or shortly thereafter. Screening is performed by feeling your child's neck to determine the size and texture of his or her thyroid gland and by performing blood tests. If your child's thyroid screen is normal, his or her medical provider might recommend repeating the screen in 1-2 years. If your child's thyroid screen is abnormal, his or her medical provider might recommend obtaining additional blood tests or starting your child on a medication to help regulate the level of thyroid hormone in the blood.

Celiac disease

Individuals with type 1 diabetes are also at an increased risk for a condition called celiac disease. Celiac disease is an immune-mediated disorder that causes damage to the small intestine and prevents the normal digestion of food. If a child has celiac disease, damage to the lining of the small intestine occurs after the child ingests a substance called gluten. Gluten is found in wheat, rye, and barley. Some refer to this condition as an allergy to wheat.

Symptoms of celiac disease include diarrhea, weight loss or poor weight gain, growth failure, abdominal pain, chronic fatigue, irritability, an inability to concentrate, malnutrition due to malabsorption, and other gastrointestinal (digestive) problems. Symptoms of celiac disease in patients who also have diabetes may include unpredictable blood glucose levels and unexplained low blood glucose reactions.

If your child has type 1 diabetes, his or her medical provider might recommend obtaining a blood test to screen your child for celiac disease. If the initial screen is abnormal, your child's medical provider will likely recommend either repeating the screen in 6-12 months or having your child seen by a gastroenterologist for further evaluation and confirmation of the diagnosis.

At present, the only treatment for celiac disease is a gluten-free diet. If your child has diabetes and celiac disease, his or her medical provider will likely recommend that you receive nutritional counseling from a registered dietitian who has experience with both conditions. A gluten-free diet means avoiding foods that contain wheat, rye, and barley. Many grocery stores and a lot of restaurants now have gluten-free items, even gluten-free pizza.

Summary

Though children with diabetes are at risk for the long-term complications of diabetes and other diabetes-health related risks, it is important to remember that our knowledge, the diabetes treatment tools, and the care available to your child today lower those risks significantly from days gone by. The most important factor in reducing the risk of future complications is to always access diabetes healthcare. Diabetes complications have early warning signs — red flags which can usually be noted and addressed by the healthcare team. Prevention, improvement, and/or stopping further progression of complications are all possibilities. Keep your child or teen engaged in diabetes care — it will set a pattern for a long and healthy life.

Web sites:

- National Diabetes education Clearinghouse: diabetes.niddk.nih.gov
- American Diabetes Association: www.diabetes.org

17

Transitions: The Challenges of Life after High School

Although leaving high school and turning 18 are traditional markers of transitioning to adulthood, no one becomes an adult overnight. Some of us take longer than others! Many factors effect how this process unfolds. Some of these factors include:

- Personality and temperament
- Developmental stage
- Level of autonomy
- Previous parental involvement and support
- How dramatically life changes after high school

The trajectory life takes after graduation often goes in one of two directions: the academic route or the working route. As a child transitions he or she will face many challenges regardless of which direction is taken, and having diabetes can add to those challenges.

The Academic Transition

So your child got into college; congratulations! Now what? First, let us look at some specific issues that should be on your child's mind as he or she is preparing to go to college. Your child may be living in a dorm, which opens a door to an entire world of unsupervised freedom that can be exciting and a little nerve-wracking as a new college student. Alternatively, your child may continue living at home and commute to school. Either way he or she is stepping into a new world where there is constantly something to do, high fat and carbohydrate foods appearing at all hours of the day and night, and a multitude of opportunities, such as intramural or informal sports and activities, taking place practically 24 hours a day. Young adults may feel like there is not enough time to take it all in and get enough time to sleep. The constant bombardment can be overwhelming if they do not learn to prioritize what is important to their college experience and remember to take care of themselves and stay healthy and yes — study.

Movin' on Out — Packing and Planning Ahead

If your child moves away from home, he or she will need to decide what to pack to take care of his or her diabetes, as well as everything else he or she will need for college. In addition to the typical school supplies, he or she will need to pack his or her usual day-to-day diabetes kit which should include:

- Insulin vials/cartridges
- Insulin syringes or insulin pens and pen needles
- Pump supplies if he or she is on an insulin pump
- Back-up pump infusion set inserter (if he or she uses an inserter)
- Blood glucose meter with:
  - strips
  - lancets
  - batteries
- Back up meter
- Blood ketone meter with strips or urine ketone strips
- Fast-acting carbohydrates to treat hypoglycemia
- Snacks
- Glucagon kit, if there is someone who can be trained at his school to give him glucagon
- Calculator to help with insulin dosing
- Mini refrigerator to store insulin (if the dorms do not come equipped with a refrigerator)

In addition to the day to day diabetes supplies he or she should also pack a sick-day kit. The sick-day kit should include the items listed in Table 17-1.

Table 17-1. Sick-Day Kit Items

• Thermometer	• A copy of your child's sick-day insulin plan
• Ketone testing supplies: » blood ketone meter and strips, or » urine ketone strips	• Your child's healthcare team's emergency contact numbers
• Nonperishable liquids like: » sports drinks » diet and non-diet soda » soup broths	
• Nonperishable bland foods like: » gelatin (sugared and sugar-free) » saltines » hard candies such as lollipops (sugared and sugar-free) » popsicles (if you have a small freezer) » bread for toast	

When your child is not feeling well he or she will want all these items in an easy to find place. He or she may never have had to handle a sick day on his or her own prior to moving away. Before he or she goes to college, have him or her review the general sick-day rules with his or her healthcare team and have a *written plan* she can refer to. Your child will need to keep in mind that basal or long-acting insulin (NPH, glargine, or detemir) is always needed to avoid developing high blood glucose and ketones due to a lack of insulin, even when he or she is not eating. If he or she has a fever, your child may have high blood glucose and ketones due to the stress hormones from the illness. For a more complete discussion of sick-day management see Chapter 11: Sick Days and DKA Prevention.

Additionally, hangovers from consuming too much alcohol can cause college students to become very sick with dehydration and vomiting. If your child is vomiting and dehydrated, he or she needs to remember to take basal or long-acting insulin, drink small amounts of fluid frequently, check his or her blood glucose every 2-3 hours, check for ketones, and call his or her diabetes healthcare team.

Finally, make sure you and your child have arranged how he or she will receive insulin and other prescriptions while at college. You may mail many of the needed prescription refills, if that is how you decide to handle them, but avoid putting insulin in the mail. If your child will not be home on a frequent basis, two additional solutions are to:

1. Make arrangements with a pharmacy near the college.
2. Use a mail order pharmacy to order insulin and any other prescriptions (make sure the mail order pharmacy will provide special packaging to keep the insulin cool).

Who to Tell?

Many young adults are nervous about moving away from the familiar. At home they have an established support system to help them manage their diabetes, and all of their friends in high school probably knew they had diabetes. People whom they knew and trusted were watching out for them everyday. Now they will have to decide who and how they should tell about their diabetes. If they are living in a dorm, their roommate and resident assistant (RA) should know that they have diabetes and should have a plan for dealing with low blood glucose levels when their blood glucose is too low for them to help themselves.

Many colleges put future roommates in contact with one another before they ever meet. If your child wants to give his roommate time to get comfortable with the idea that he has diabetes he could introduce the topic before he gets to school. This can allow time to make adjustments or arrangements if needed. On the other hand, he may choose to wait until he meets his roommate and discuss this face-to-face. A safe way to practice discussing this topic is for your child to ask his current friends if they have any suggestions as to how your child might introduce that fact that he has diabetes to a new roommate and friends at college. The staff at the college health center should know that your child has diabetes. Finally, even if your child tells a few people that he has diabetes, there will still be many students and staff at his college who do not know this. Your child should always wear a medical alert bracelet or necklace. Having a back up medical alert wallet card is a helpful, though less reliable, alternative to a medical alert necklace or bracelet.

Hypoglycemia

If your child is living on campus and has a roommate, he or she will want to bring up the issue of hypoglycemia. Low blood glucose levels tend to occur more frequently at night early on in college, especially with the increase in late night activities and exercise, frequent late night snacking with more insulin being given late at night, and increased exposure to alcohol. Your child needs to be careful about covering large amounts of carbohydrates with insulin late at night before going to sleep. Large doses of rapid-acting insulin can last longer than he or she expects and can cause low blood glucose levels. If your child has a roommate, his or her roommate should know that if he or she wakes up at night and appears to be confused or is having a nightmare, that this could be a sign of a low blood glucose and that the roommate should get him or her a juice or glucose gel, or whatever his or her standard treatment of choice is for hypoglycemia. In the event of a seizure or loss of consciousness, your child's roommate should call 911 for professional help or have the RA do so.

Guidelines and state laws may determine who can give a glucagon injection. Check with your college health service to determine who can be taught how to inject glucagon. If it is appropriate and your child's RA, roommate, or a friend in the dorm feels comfortable learning how to give glucagon, and he or she feels comfortable asking them to give it in case of a severe episode of hypoglycemia, he or she can teach them how they would administer it. It is likely that someone who has never given an injection would find it difficult to give glucagon in an emergency. Thus, a practical alternative may be a tube of glucose gel which can be given to a semi-conscious individual who is able to swallow. Your child should also discuss with his or her roommate that some foods, such as fast-acting carbohydrates and certain snacks, are like medication and it is important that they not be eaten by others.

Storing Diabetes Supplies

Your child should try to be organized with his or her diabetes supplies. Many people who are not used to syringes find them unsettling and so your child would want to be respectful of his or her roommate's feelings, and be careful not to leave used syringes lying around. To be courteous and safe, sharps, such as syringes and lancets, should be immediately placed in a sharps container. These can be purchased in some pharmacies. A detergent container is also a reasonable alternative. When the bottle is three-quarters full of sharps, the cap should be secured by taping it with duct tape. It can then be brought home for disposal, according to local trash regulations. Some states require labeled sharps containers for disposal of sharps. Your child may also want to consider keeping syringes in a locked box in a drawer or in an under-the-bed storage container with his or her other diabetes supplies. Locked boxes are available in office supply stores.

Eating at College

Navigating food choices in college can be tricky. Scheduling a nutrition visit with your child's dietitian to review carbohydrate counting the summer before starting college is highly recommended. If your child does not know how to carbohydrate count, it is advisable for him or her to learn before leaving home. When your child is eating away from home, nutritional content information may not be readily available. Obtaining it is often not difficult, but it does require a little additional effort on your child's part. If he or she will be eating in a cafeteria, there should be a member of the food services staff who can assist in finding the nutritional information that he or she needs. Many colleges try to accommodate students with special dietary needs, such as diabetes, celiac disease, or religious needs. If your child is not able to find the nutritional information of something new that he or she is eating, he or she can also try checking his or her blood glucose two hours after eating the meal to see how he or she is doing with the carbohydrate counting estimate, and to see if any insulin adjustments are needed. Also, portion control can be very difficult in a cafeteria because the food is often presented in an all-you-can-eat buffet style, so your child will want to try to remember to eat in moderation. If your child is not living in a dorm and is cooking on his or her own for the first time, he or she may also want to talk to the cook in your family or meet with a dietitian before leaving for college to learn how to prepare some simple healthy meals.

Blood Glucose Fluctuations

In addition to all the late night events that can cause unexpected blood glucose levels, the increase in the amount of walking on campus, the unlimited cafeteria style eating, and the overall change in routine can also cause high and low blood glucose fluctuations that your child is not accustomed to managing. Monitoring your child's blood glucose more frequently (at least 4 times a day) is very important as he or she makes the transition to a new lifestyle away from home. Logbooks can be a nuisance to keep, but they are very helpful for recognizing patterns. Your child can also get programs to download the blood glucoses and information in his meter or pump into his computer instead of keeping a logbook on paper. If he recognizes a pattern of erratic blood glucoses, he should contact his diabetes healthcare team to make adjustments in his insulin program if needed; it does not make sense for your child to struggle with blood glucose numbers on his own until the next visit with his regular diabetes healthcare team, when they are available to assist him by telephone or email.

College Health Center and Services

As a student in a new environment, your child should take the time to learn where and how to access the available support systems at his or her college, which usually includes college health and counseling services and student diabetes support groups. As previously stated, when accessing services at the college health center, or really anywhere that his or her history is not previously known, it is especially important for your child to tell the medical staff that he or she has diabetes. The medical form that your child had completed by his or her healthcare provider should be kept in a place designated by the school Healthcare Services or Infirmary.

Diabetic Ketoacidosis

Diabetic ketoacidosis, or DKA, can present with similar symptoms to many other vomiting illnesses that affect college-age students. If your child is sick, he or she will need to take an active role in checking blood glucoses and ketones and recognize that what might appear to be an intestinal virus with vomiting may be ketoacidosis. Your child's college infirmary can be very helpful if he or she is ill, but their clinicians may not be experts in diabetes management. Before leaving for school, your child will want to discuss with his or her diabetes healthcare team where back up diabetes-related care can be sought near the college if needed. If he or she does end up at the college infirmary, the infirmary staff may also want to talk to his or her diabetes healthcare team if there are questions about diabetes management during illness.

Health Insurance

Whether working or a full-time student (and at some schools if your child is a three-quarter time student), he or she may be eligible to remain on your health insurance policy. If that is not an option, many colleges and employers offer affordable health insurance to students or individuals younger than 25 years old. So if your child is facing a change in health insurance coverage, or he or she does not have health insurance coverage, it is important to explore all available options and to carefully read the policies being offered. For example, your child will want to pick a plan that has good prescription coverage. Your child needs health insurance coverage; he or she should make sure to look at all of the options.

The Working Transition

If your child decides to work instead of going to college, there are a few different issues that need to be considered. From a legal standpoint, during an interview, your child does not have to disclose that he or she has diabetes, and an employer cannot ask if he or she has diabetes or uses insulin or other prescription drugs. If your child does disclose that she has diabetes during an interview, the employer is only allowed to ask two questions: whether she needs a reasonable accommodation because she has diabetes and what type of accommodation she will need.

If your child decides to withhold the fact that he or she has diabetes until after accepting a position, then he or she will have to make the decision as to how to approach the topic with his or her employer once he or she starts working. Remember that the employer must provide reasonable accommodations in order for your child to manage his or her diabetes. The Americans with Disabilities Act is an excellent resource to learn more about what constitutes reasonable accommodations (see http://www.ada.gov/). Finally, your child will also need to decide if he or she wants to disclose to co-workers that he or she has diabetes. Regardless of his or her decisions, a medical alert bracelet or necklace should always be worn so appropriate actions can be taken to get help in an emergency.

Finding the balance of being able to care for and appropriately manage diabetes in the context of a new job is very important. If your child's blood glucose is low he or she may make errors in calculations, judgment, or have trouble performing the tasks of his or her job. If your child's job involves using machine tools or driving, low blood glucoses can put him or her at special risk of injury. If his or her blood glucose is high, your child may have difficulty concentrating, or be tired and irritable, which can make him or her difficult to work with. Additionally, long-term high blood glucose values can negatively affect his or her ability to perform his job day-to-day. Taking better care of him- or herself increases the potential to be a better performing employee.

When starting a job, your child should discuss health insurance options with the Human Resources department to learn what kind of benefits are offered, and to review the different policies carefully to insure that he or she is choosing the best plan offered to suit his or her needs. It is also worth finding out when his or her health insurance coverage begins and deciding if he or she needs to find a temporary plan that allows coverage until that time. Sometimes there is a delay before health insurance coverage begins following being hired.

In the event of a job change, your child can ask the Human Resources department if COBRA insurance is available. COBRA stands for the Consolidated Omnibus Budget Reconciliation Act, and is a temporary continuation of health insurance coverage. It can be expensive, but for people with diabetes, it might be a necessity.

Working may involve your child living at home or venturing out into his or her own apartment. Much of what has been said about dorm life would apply if yoiur child is moving out of your family home. Apartments don't come with a cafeteria, but fast food may substitute for home cooked meals. If your child's trash can shows that the majority of his or her meals came from a delivery or drive through, it is time for him or her to consider learning how to cook simple healthy meals. Apartment living right out of high school typically means roommates and the section above regarding roommates is applicable whether your child is in college or working.

Diabetes and Tobacco, Drug and Alcohol Use

Whether your child takes the academic or working route, it is important for him or her to know how tobacco, drug, and alcohol use can affect his or her diabetes. Your child has probably heard that smoking, drinking, and drug use are unhealthy, but it is important for him or her to know what happens to his or her body if he or she does use these substances. First off, it is worth starting this discussion with the obvious. It is illegal to purchase or use cigarettes under the age of 18, it is illegal to purchase or use alcohol under the age of 21, and it is always illegal to purchase or use any illegal drugs. Drug and alcohol use in general poses two very large risks related to diabetes management. Drugs and alcohol can impair judgment and they mask symptoms of hypoglycemia and hyperglycemia. The actual effect of a particular drug on a person is widely variable because they are made illegally without standards or controls. It is very important for your child to monitor his or her blood glucose frequently if he or she is using any of the substances listed in this section.

Tobacco

Tobacco use is a concern in teens and young adults because tobacco contains nicotine which is highly addictive for everyone. The tobacco companies recognize the young adult population as vulnerable potential future clients and advertise their products near many college campuses with free promotional items, including packs of cigarettes. While tobacco use has been proven harmful for everyone, smoking can be especially dangerous for people with diabetes. High blood glucose levels can stress the body's small blood vessels over time and nicotine in cigarettes and other tobacco products speeds up this damage by narrowing blood vessels, which can lead to eye disease, kidney disease, and impotence, and increases the risk of high blood pressure, heart attacks, and stroke.

Alcohol

The liver has many responsibilities in the body, including the manufacture, storage, and release of glycogen (stored sugar). When your child consumes alcohol, the functions of the liver are impaired, because the liver has to try to rid the body of the toxins in the alcohol. This can cause rapid and/or delayed hypoglycemia, which can persist for hours after alcohol consumption. Symptoms of high and low blood glucose can be similar to the symptoms of intoxication, so individuals who are intoxicated may not appropriately recognize and treat low or high blood glucose. If your child goes to a party, drinks a lot of alcohol, perhaps exercises by dancing, and falls asleep intoxicated, he can have an unconscious hypoglycemic reaction with a seizure during the night or the next morning. Others at the party may not realize that one of the people sleeping it off actually is unconscious due to hypoglycemia. A drinking binge can lead to a trip to the closest emergency department for intravenous glucose and fluids. This does not happen every time people drink large amounts of alcohol, so people get fooled into thinking it will not happen to them.

Managing blood glucose levels can be very tricky with alcohol. In order to cover up the taste of the alcohol, many drinks are mixed with very sweet, high carbohydrate-content liquids, which can cause very high blood glucose levels. These highs early in an evening, combined with the low blood glucose that can result from alcohol consumption later on, can make managing blood glucose levels very hard. In addition, if your child drinks too much alcohol, he or she puts him- or herself at risk for alcohol poisoning, which may cause vomiting that night or the next morning. Vomiting increases the risk for developing ketones, which can get your child into trouble quickly.

There is no safe way to drink alcohol. Since alcohol impairs judgment, people can make poor decisions under the influence of alcohol. They may make poor choices about diabetes management, as well as poor decisions about sexual activity, driving, and other risky choices. We recommend that young adults do not use alcohol. Some teens and young adults have told us that they like using their diabetes as an excuse not to drink alcohol when they are experiencing peer pressure.

If your child is going to drink, the following guidelines will reduce his or her risk of alcohol induced hypoglycemia and help keep him or her safer:

- Stay with a friend who knows he has diabetes.
- Have fast-acting carbohydrate treatments with him.

- Eat before consuming alcohol to avoid drinking on an empty stomach.
- Alternate alcoholic beverages with water or other non alcoholic beverages andlimit the intake to 1-2 drinks over the course of the entire evening (1 drink is a 12 oz beer, 4 oz wine, 1 oz of alcohol in a mixed drink).
  - 1 drink per evening for women
  - 1-2 drinks per evening for men
- Drink slowly and avoid chugging alcohol or consuming shots of liquor, which can cause alcohol poisoning.
- Monitor blood glucose frequently, especially when dancing or exercising.
- Wear a medical alert bracelet or necklace.
- Set an alarm clock to check blood glucose in the middle of the night, before going out.
- Discuss insulin adjustments for specific situations with his diabetes healthcare team.
- Never drink and drive.

Drugs

As drugs are illegal, damaging to the body, and dangerous, no advice can be given for their usage. Here we will provide some facts about how they can negatively impact diabetes.

- Marijuana use can be problematic because marijuana stimulates appetite and impairs judgment. This can lead to poor decision-making about overeating and diabetes management, which can cause high blood glucose levels. It also causes problems with short-term memory, concentration, problem solving, and sensory and time perception, which can all negatively affect blood glucose control. Frequent marijuana use can lead to addiction and Amotivational Syndrome, a lack of energy and direction, which severely impairs college or job performance.
- Cocaine constricts blood vessels while increasing blood pressure, which increases the risk of heart attack or stroke. Cocaine can decrease appetite and the effects of cocaine can mask or

imitate symptoms of low blood glucose. Cocaine use is also a risk factor for diabetic ketoacidosis.
- Psychedelics alter one's perception of reality which can make it very difficult to manage diabetes.
  - Ecstasy can produce the feeling of endless energy. Ecstasy is often taken at raves or dance parties where users can be very active and distracted, making a person with diabetes unaware of his or her usual low blood glucose symptoms. This in turn can lead to dehydration and severe hypoglycemia. Repeated use of ecstasy can cause chemical depression.
  - Opiates, oxycontin and heroin use are extremely addictive and can alter perception, decrease energy and can change eating habits. Opiates and heroin are extremely dangerous due to the risk of unintentional overdose.

Sexual Health

It is vital for women with diabetes to avoid unplanned pregnancy. Blood glucoses need to be monitored very closely before becoming pregnant and during pregnancy to decrease the risk of birth defects. Women who are interested in becoming pregnant should talk to their diabetes team about following an intensive insulin regimen appropriate for becoming pregnant. There are a number of effective contraceptive methods available and women who are sexually active but do not want to become pregnant should use contraception, which often includes an oral contraceptive pill (birth control pill) and condoms. Condom use is recommended for both men and women to prevent the transmission of sexually transmitted diseases.

Keeping in mind that sexual activity is a form of exercise, a source of fast-acting carbohydrates should be available to prevent or treat hypoglycemia. Additionally, just like other form of activity, checking blood glucose before and after sexual activity will help to maintain control of blood glucose.

Health Care

As a young adult with diabetes, it is important that your child know where and how to access healthcare. This includes access to primary and preventative care, urgent care, diabetes-related care, and mental health and counseling as needed. Primary care well visits, as well as gynecological services for women, should be scheduled annually. Diabetes care visits should be scheduled every 3 months, and nutrition and eye exams should be scheduled annually. Mental health services should be scheduled as needed.

Your child should discuss with his or her primary care provider whether he or she is up-to-date with immunizations. Many, if not all colleges require the routine pediatric vaccinations. Additionally, if your child is living on campus, he or she may need the meningococcal vaccine, and certain academic majors or study abroad programs may require further vaccinations. If your child is working, some positions require routine pediatric vaccinations as well. Some vaccinations given in childhood, such as the tetanus and diphtheria vaccine, require a booster in adulthood to remain effective. The pneumococcal vaccine is appropriate for people with diabetes. Women who have not yet had a human papilloma virus vaccine series should discuss this with their provider.

Current Diabetes Management Plan

It is important for your child to recognize how these upcoming changes and transitions can and will affect his or her current diabetes management plan. The insulin dosing, schedule, or form of insulin administration that he or she used in high school may not be appropriate in young adulthood. For greater flexibility, many young adults change to a basal/bolus insulin regimen via pump therapy or with once-daily long-acting basal insulin and rapid-acting bolus insulin for meals and high blood glucose values. Going to college or working may involve dramatic changes in your child's schedule, making it much less routine than high school. Any job that involves rotating between day and night shifts can present its own set of challenges that should be discussed with your child's diabetes healthcare team.

It is also important for your child to think about how his or her eating and physical activity may change. He or she may be eating away from home more and may need to make insulin adjustments accordingly. Opportunities for physical fitness may increase or decrease depending on campus or community resources, his or her motivation to be active, and how much time he or she has in his or her new schedule. Healthy, well-balanced meals and regular physical activity at least 5 days per week for 30 minutes is strongly recommended. If you or your child suspect any disordered eating behaviors, these behaviors should be addressed immediately. It is important for your child to find a balance between his or her academic or professional life, social life, and his or her health.

Transitioning to Adult Medicine

No matter which direction your child's life is heading as a young adult with diabetes, his or her diabetes healthcare team should be an ever-present support system. Different pediatric diabetes programs transition patients to an adult provider at different ages. Some pediatric programs transition patients to adult care at age 19, but many centers encourage young adults to stay with their pediatric team through their early 20s. Graduating from high school does not mean that your child's pediatric team is no longer appropriate. Having a long-standing relationship with a familiar and trusted medical team can help ease the transitions that he or she faces in young adulthood. The transition process can proceed gradually over several years. Pediatric providers work hard over the years to support your child and your family and it would be irresponsible to discontinue care during this transition period. Over multiples visits, your child and his or her diabetes healthcare team can discuss how to facilitate the future transition, as well as his or her choices for adult care providers and facilities. Pediatric providers can often offer assistance in identifying adult providers who might best meet the patient's needs.

When choosing an adult diabetes specialist, consider the following factors:

- How many young adults do they see in their practice?
- Do they enjoy working with young adults?

- Do they have the expertise to address the issues of:
  - heart and blood vessel health
  - management of high blood pressure
  - elevated cholesterol levels
  - neuropathy
  - sexual function
  - preparing for pregnancy

Independent health behaviors are an important part of beginning the transition to adult medicine. Before making an appointment, your child should be introduced to the referral process and how to obtain any needed referrals. He or she should gather important information, such as the names of his or her medications with doses and instructions, and what medications need to be refilled. Your child should also gather any pertinent previous health information, such as lab results, or a documented menstrual cycle pattern. He or she may want to have her pediatric medical record transferred to the new adult provider. We also suggest that your child write down any questions that he or she has ahead of time to bring to the next appointment. Adult visits may be briefer than pediatric ones so that is why it is important to be prepared and bring blood glucose monitoring data with him or her and to think ahead about special questions or goals for diabetes management he or she would like to address during the visit.

On the appointment day, your child should bring his or her written questions, insurance card, blood glucose logbook, meter or meter downloads, and any updated health information that he or she has gathered. You, as a parent, are encouraged to support your child in this process, but your child should start to take charge of some of these tasks.

During an appointment, your child should expect to see his or her diabetes specialist without a parent or guardian in the exam room, ask questions, and know his or her own diabetes treatment plan, including:

- Medications and doses
- Current insulin plan
- How often he is checking his blood glucose

Your child should also know how to contact his or her diabetes healthcare team if he or she has any questions, concerns, or problems after the visit.

At the end of a visit your child should learn how to schedule his or her next follow-up appointment and how to get a referral if needed for additional medical services. Your child also may need to learn how to arrange transportation to his or her visits if he or she is no longer going to visits with a parent or family member. Finally, your child should know how to fill or refill his or her prescriptions.

How Parents Can Stay Involved and Encourage Support Systems

Legally, a teen becomes an adult at age 18. Emotionally, becoming an adult can take years. Even though your teen may be an adult legally, it does not eliminate the important role that you play as a parent. Many young adults still want and need you to help them with their diabetes management. However, when your child is 18 years old, the Health Insurance Portability and Accountability Act (HIPAA) restricts you from any medical information regarding your young adult son or daughter. If your child wants you to remain involved in his or her medical care, medical releases should be signed by your child, who should clarify what medical information can be discussed with you, such as updates to his or her diabetes management plan and lab values. For many college students, keeping you in the loop with their diabetes care is essential. You may be included in part of the visit and discussions, as they desire.

Parents can help prepare young adults during these transitions by encouraging them to take a more active and autonomous role in their diabetes management. Some specific suggestions include:

- Make sure your child understands his or her diabetes management plan.
- Make sure your child knows how to count carbohydrates without your assistance.
- Make sure your child understands sick-day rules.
- Make sure your child knows how to fill or refill a prescription.

- Teach your child how to make an appointment.
- Help your child with possible roadblocks, such as obtaining referrals and dealing with other insurance issues.

There are ways for parents to help their college-aged sons or daughters when they are off at school. Parents can schedule their medical appointments for school vacations; check in with them regularly when they are at school to see how they are doing; ask their children if they have enough diabetes supplies and, if they are running out of supplies, remind them to order prescriptions and diabetes supplies locally, by mail or help them by mailing supplies to them. College students love to receive packages, so you could also send your son or daughter fast-acting carbohydrates and healthy snacks that he or she likes. That new apartment dweller, non-cook, would love a home cooked meal too!

Try to remember that your young adult son or daughter expects that you will ask about his or her diabetes, as you always have; but when speaking with him or her over the phone or computer, it should not be the first question that you ask. Teens and young adults with diabetes do not define themselves by their diabetes. In clinic, we often recommend a 3-question minimum — suggesting that you discuss 3 topics unrelated to diabetes before asking about blood glucose numbers or other diabetes-related issues.

Parents should encourage your young adult son or daughter to explore their interests further in college, at work, or in community-based activities. If your child enjoyed sports in high school, but is not pursuing competitive collegiate level athletics, there may be another way for your child to remain active. Many schools and workplaces offer club and intramural sports or have gyms to work out.

Most colleges have non-athletic organizations that your child may be interested in, such as academic organizations, international and multicultural clubs, religious groups, music and performing arts clubs, environmental organizations, political groups, student governments, social service clubs, and fraternities and sororities. Most towns and cities have community-based sports teams, religious organizations that support social organizations, music ensembles and symphonies, as well as groups such as BigBrother/BigSister, etc. Many colleges are developing student-run diabetes social networks that your child may be interested in joining.

Finally, young adults and their parents are encouraged to explore local support services where they will be living and/or attending school. Young adults who appear socially isolated, anxious or depressed should receive counseling and support services prior to leaving for college and arrangements should be made for services to continue while at school.

Some Final Thoughts

The transition years from the end of high school through the twenties are an exciting and challenging time for young adults with diabetes. Maturation of judgment and self esteem continue throughout these years. Diabetes management may not always be optimal as young adults make the transition to full independence. The most important goal for your child as a young adult and for you is to keep up regular visits with a diabetes healthcare team during these years, including yearly visits for eye exams. Your child needs to find a diabetes care provider who he or she can learn to work with honestly and comfortably. Your child will gradually figure out how to fit diabetes into his or her adult life and work toward becoming an expert in managing his or her own diabetes with the help of family and the right diabetes care team.

References and Resources

Gilliland A, Siminerio L. . For parents. Getting ready for college. *Diabetes Self-Management*. 2002;19(1):88, 91-2, 94, 96.

Glick, D. Legal and illegal drugs: what every person with diabetes should know before they party. *Diabetes Health*. Nov 2003. Available at: http://www.diabeteshealth.com/read/2008/03/13/3163.html.

The U.S. Equal Employment Opportunity Commission. Questions and answers about diabetes in the workplace and the Americans with Disabilities Act (ADA). The U.S. Equal Employment Opportunity Commission Website. 2003. Available at: http://www.eeoc.gov/facts/diabetes.html.

18

New Technologies and Current Research

At the Joslin Diabetes Center, caring for and curing diabetes remains our mission. This chapter will highlight recent advances and new directions in diabetes technologies and research. The speed and diversity of technological advances continue in the 21st century. Management of pediatric type 1 diabetes, utilizing emerging technologies, creates an exciting time for both families and healthcare providers. Better technology assists treatment by mimicking normal insulin production, and gives a means to improve blood glucose control. Families and kids with diabetes, today, have an increasing number of tools to better achieve intensive management with improved quality of life, more flexibility, and fewer burdens. As an example, just since 1996, 5 new insulins have become available for pediatric use.

Type 1 diabetes research continues with a cure and its prevention as the ultimate goal. The current menu of research is extensive in scope and practice. ClinicalTrials.gov, a service of the U.S. National Institutes of Health, lists over 450 type 1 diabetes studies. Studies are ongoing, investigating such topics as stem cells, oral insulin, exercise, pump therapy, telemedicine and cinnamon! Research is broad and far reaching, from the test tube to animals to genetic research, and includes many human trials.

In this chapter we will review what is *new* and different and what is in the technology pipeline in the following areas:

- Glucose monitoring, including continuous monitoring
- Point of care A1C testing
- Insulin
- Insulin delivery systems, including insulin pumps
- Genetic testing

- Electronic telecommunications
- Type 1 research

Glucose Monitoring

Self-monitoring of blood glucose (BG) is one tool that helps to self-manage diabetes on a daily basis. There are a variety of available meters today for self-monitoring of BG. What new features do specific meters have that are different in 2009?

- Larger buttons
- No coding or automatic coding
- Strip ejector
- Audio feature (also available in Spanish)
- A meter that is also a cell phone
- Wireless transmission of data

For more details go to: http://forecast.diabetes.org/magazine/resource-guide/2009-resource-guide.

Continuous Glucose Monitoring

BG meters provide what is called episodic information. They do not provide continuous readings or information on the rate and direction of change in blood glucose concentration. Continuous Glucose Monitoring (CGM) is a relatively recent technological advance that provides *real-time* blood glucose data every 1-5 minutes, allowing the person with diabetes and his or her healthcare provider to track glucose levels throughout the day. We need to be clear, though, that CGM does not replace blood glucose checking with a meter; it supplements this information to give you a better understanding of what is happening to glucose levels. The FDA approved CGM devices are described in Chapter 6: Monitoring Glucose and Ketones. Please refer to that chapter to learn about their components and how they work.

Each year brings upgrades to the technology. This technology provides detailed information about glucose fluctuations: extent, duration, frequency of low and high glucose levels, relationship of excursions in glucose to certain activities or foods, and trend data to help the individual predict and possibly prevent hyper or hypoglycemia. In addition, CGM is the first step in closing the loop for an artificial pancreas.

Questions regarding the safety, accuracy, and psychological impact of continuous glucose monitors in the pediatric population remain. It is possible that CGM will reduce anxiety about hypoglycemia, but it may also increase anxiety when the continuous glucose monitor data and the results from traditional self-monitoring do not agree. In addition, the amount of glucose data may overwhelm you and your child and increase the burden of diabetes management. The Diabetes Research in Children Network (DirecNet) Study Group recently published data on the psychological outcomes from a randomized trial of the GlucoWatch G2 Biographer. Results from surveys measuring diabetes treatment adherence, diabetes-specific quality of life, and diabetes-related anxiety demonstrated that there were no adverse or beneficial psychological effects of CGM using the GlucoWatch G2 Biographer. However, the GlucoWatch differs enough from the other currently available technologies that the results from this trial may not be transferable to newer sensors. A recent study funded by the Juvenile Diabetes Research Foundation (JDRF) demonstrated significant benefit of CGM in adults with type 1 diabetes and found similar benefits of CGM technologies in youth with type 1 diabetes who wore the devices consistently.

The iPro is a new continuous monitoring device that is inserted by a member of a healthcare team and does not provide real-time data. It is not purchased by the patient or his or her family; rather it is owned by the diabetes center. It takes a reading every 5 minutes over 72 hours, but does not provide any real-time data. The glucose levels are hidden in the device until it is returned to the healthcare team for downloading. The hidden data from the iPro are downloaded directly to a computer for review by the healthcare team. This gives the diabetes team a wealth of information to help in making changes to the diabetes management plan.

Point of Care A1C Testing

A1C is the gold standard for evaluating glycemic control. The healthcare provider's knowledge of a person's A1C helps to manage diabetes and improve metabolic control. Point of care testing of A1C (done in a laboratory or your healthcare provider's office) offers immediate results that

Table 18-1. A1C Translation to eAG

Average glucose = (28.7 x A1C) – 46.7

A1C (%)	Average Glucose (mg/dL)	A1C (%)	Average Glucose (mg/dL)	A1C (%)	Average Glucose (mg/dL)	A1C (%)	Average Glucose (mg/dL)
5.0	97	8.0	183	11.0	269	14.0	355
5.1	100	8.1	186	11.1	272	14.1	358
5.2	103	8.2	189	11.2	275	14.2	361
5.3	105	8.3	192	11.3	278	14.3	364
5.4	108	8.4	194	11.4	280	14.4	367
5.5	111	8.5	197	11.5	283	14.5	369
5.6	114	8.6	200	11.6	286	14.6	372
5.7	117	8.7	203	11.7	289	14.7	375
5.8	120	8.8	206	11.8	292	14.8	378
5.9	123	8.9	209	11.9	295	14.9	381
6.0	126	9.0	212	12.0	298	15.0	384
6.1	128	9.1	214	12.1	301	15.1	387
6.2	131	9.2	217	12.2	303	15.2	390
6.3	134	9.3	220	12.3	306	15.3	392
6.4	137	9.4	223	12.4	309	15.4	395
6.5	140	9.5	226	12.5	312	15.5	398
6.6	143	9.6	229	12.6	315	15.6	401
6.7	146	9.7	232	12.7	318	15.7	404
6.8	148	9.8	235	12.8	321	15.8	407
6.9	151	9.9	237	12.9	324	15.9	410
7.0	154	10.0	240	13.0	326	16.0	413
7.1	157	10.1	243	13.1	329		
7.2	160	10.2	246	13.2	332		
7.3	163	10.3	249	13.3	335		
7.4	166	10.4	252	13.4	338		
7.5	169	10.5	255	13.5	341		
7.6	171	10.6	258	13.6	344		
7.7	174	10.7	260	13.7	346		
7.8	177	10.8	263	13.8	349		
7.9	180	10.9	266	13.9	352		

can confirm the accuracy of BG monitoring data. Additionally, the immediate A1C result may be all that is available if you forget to bring your meters or logbooks. An immediate A1C result at the visit helps direct therapy changes aimed at improving blood glucose control.

Studies in adults show that the point of care A1C assay results in significant improvement of blood glucose control at 6- and 12-month follow-up visits. A recent study used point of care A1C testing compared with A1C laboratory measurements in the evaluation of active versus usual titration of insulin on glycemic control. While these studies involved adults with diabetes, children with diabetes, their families, and providers alike are also expected to benefit from immediate point of care A1C testing. In turn, any improvement in A1C levels for children will lead to a reduction or postponement in the development of diabetes complications. As an added benefit, children will appreciate the opportunity to avoid venipuncture (blood drawn from the arm) with point of care A1C testing, which is obtained by finger stick.

The A1C test will continue to be done; however, as discussed in Chapter 6: Monitoring Glucose and Ketones, the eAG (estimated Average Glucose) is a new way to present the same information in numbers more like the ones you see on your child's blood glucose meter. The American Diabetes Association has an eAG calculator available at: http://www.diabetes.org/eag.jsp. Table 18-1 shows how an A1C will be translated from a percentage to a blood glucose value — the eAG.

Insulin

Insulin analogues have been developed by biochemically altering the human insulin molecule, thereby modifying its time to onset, peak activity, and duration of action. The first analogue was approved by the FDA in 1996. Since then, 4 other insulin analogues have been approved.

For additional information on available insulins, see Chapter 4: Insulin.

Insulin Delivery Systems

There are some newer options for insulin delivery. Insulin pens have become increasingly popular among pediatric patients and their families because they appear more discreet than vials of insulin and syringes, and are more convenient and portable. Some pens are reusable, others are disposable. Most types of rapid-acting, intermediate-acting, long-acting, and mixed insulin preparations are available in pens. Proper use of insulin pens requires education for children and caregivers on topics such as:

- Storage
- Gentle rolling of pens that contain NPH prior to use
- Removing needle tips in-between doses to prevent insulin leakage and air entry
- Adequate priming of the pen to ensure accurate dosing
- Holding the pen in place for several seconds after injection to avoid leakage

There is even a new pen with a memory. More information is available at: forecast.diabetes.org/files/images/InsulinPenChart.pdf. Some pens are pediatric friendly and allow dosing insulin in increments of 0.5 units.

Insulin Infusers

Most children and adolescents tolerate injections very well, with minimal discomfort; however, there is a small group of patients who have heightened anxiety from needle phobia and injection pain. For such patients there are 2 insulin infusers that stay in the skin for up to 3-5 days. Once the catheter is in place, all insulin doses can be delivered via syringe or pen needle through the catheter. One study found a decrease in injection pain and anxiety in the group using indwelling catheters when compared to the control group receiving standard injections with insulin pens. A local anesthetic, such as EMLA Cream or Pain Ease Spray, can be applied prior to insertion. Additional information on insulin infusers can be found at: forecast.diabetes.org/files/images/InsulinInfusersChart.pdf.

Insulin Pumps

Use of continuous subcutaneous insulin infusion (CSII), otherwise known as insulin pump therapy, is increasing in the pediatric diabetes population. Insulin pumps deliver a continuous infusion of insulin throughout the day that mimics the basal insulin production by the pancreas. Boluses of insulin are given throughout the day to cover meals and snacks, using insulin-to-carbohydrate ratios, and to lower a glucose back to the target range, using a correction dose or sensitivity factor. With the exception of the OmniPod, which offers an integrated infusion set, automated cannula inserter, and insulin reservoir with tubeless insulin delivery, all other insulin pumps on the market are connected by thin plastic tubing to the insertion set which is inserted into the subcutaneous tissue and left in place for 2-3 days. Though insulin pumps are not new technology, a lot of the recent upgrades, such as CGM capabilities, data storage, download ability, nutrition databases, and programmable reminders, offer a way for insulin pump therapy to help families to achieve their diabetes management goals.

Company websites provide the most up-to-date information on specific features for each pump. These web sites have been provided in Chapter 5: Insulin Pumps. In addition to these sites, the following websites are also good sources of information on insulin pumps:

- DiabetesNet: www.diabetesnet.com/diabetes_technology/insulin pumps.php
- Children with Diabetes: www.childrenwithdiabetes.com/pumps/index.htm
- Insulin Pumpers: www.insulin-pumpers.org.

Electronic Communication and Tele-Health Tools

The therapeutic advances in diabetes management — new designer insulins, insulin delivery systems, and monitoring technologies — are matched by advances in information transfer and communication for families and their diabetes healthcare teams. Paper logbooks may contain incorrectly recorded data or there may be no data at all to share with the team. Use of electronic logbooks may help overcome such problems. At Joslin Diabetes Center, a study looked at blood glucose monitors with paper logbooks compared to an integrated blood glucose monitor and electronic log. There were 205 adult and pediatric insulin-treated patients in the study. After 16 weeks, the group using the electronic log had a greater decrease in average A1C compared with the paper logbook group. Furthermore, only those patients who consistently used the integrated meter with electronic log maintained their improvement in A1C over time. The electronic logbook may reduce some of the burden of diabetes since recording results is not necessary — the logbook in the monitor saves all of the information. In fact, people using the integrated meter and electronic log checked blood glucose levels more frequently, which may have provided important additional information to guide treatments to improve glucose control.

Recognizing the importance of frequent BG monitoring, Joslin Diabetes Center researchers designed an automated reminder system for adolescents and young adults with type 1 diabetes. Their system sent either email or cell phone text message reminders to check blood glucose levels at patient-selected times throughout the day. Forty 12-25 year old youths were randomly (by chance) assigned to receive email or cell phone text message reminders for 12 weeks. During the first month, nearly twice as many blood glucose checks were sent to the secure central sever where the blood glucose data were stored by the group receiving cell text message reminders. However, system usage decreased in both groups over time. This study and others support the ease with which teens and young adults with type 1 diabetes are willing to accept new technologies, but additional challenges remain in order to keep them using the systems to best manage their blood glucose levels over time.

A recently published study reported on a new tele-health initiative that can help youth better manage their diabetes. In this study 27 high-risk youths with type 1 diabetes with recurrent diabetic ketoacidosis or A1C values greater than 9% were provided psychology services and support through videophone and telephone conferencing while in the school setting. In this group there was an average A1C reduction of 0.7%. Additionally, there were no diabetes-associated hospitalizations during the study. These findings are encouraging. Additional controlled clinical studies of tele-health interventions are needed to show us the effectiveness and cost-effectiveness of these innovative approaches.

Another technological innovation in communication is the use of internet-based chat rooms and bulletin boards which provide support for children with diabetes and their families. Examples of such communication vehicles can be found at the websites of Children with Diabetes (www.childrenwithdiabetes.com/chat/) and Joslin Diabetes Center (www.joslin.org/1863.asp).

Islet Cell Transplantation

The Edmonton Protocol brought significant enthusiasm for freedom from insulin treatment for people with type 1 diabetes. The first 7 patients who received islet cell transplants using steroid-free immunosuppression were able to stop taking insulin. Due to such results, an international effort to implement the Edmonton protocol began. A recent report of 36 patients enrolled in the protocol showed that less than half had successfully achieved adequate glucose control without insulin after one year. However, 58% had become insulin independent at some point during the study. While the Edmonton protocol has advanced the field of islet transplantation in general, this approach is reserved for adults with disabling, difficult to control hypoglycemia.

Genetic Screening for Neonatal Diabetes

Another striking advance in the management of youth with insulin-treated diabetes stems from the revelation of the genetic basis of neonatal diabetes. With investigators from around the world working together, enough cases of neonatal diabetes have led to the discovery of a single gene defect as the cause of neonatal diabetes.

As a result of this finding, people with neonatal diabetes, treated with insulin for many years, in fact for decades in some instances, have been successfully transitioned from insulin therapy to oral agent therapy with improvement in glycemic control. This remarkable finding has generated the recommendation to screen all newborns and infants, developing diabetes within the first 6 months of life, for these mutations so that positive cases can be treated readily with a pill rather than with insulin. Specialized laboratories are needed for these evaluations.

Also On the Horizon:

Under development is an automated pen delivery system for glucagon. It is a little larger than an Epi-pen and there is an automated two-step process to deliver the glucagon. One step will dissolve the glucagon and a second step delivers the drug. Ask your provider for more information when it becomes available.

Artificial Pancreas System (APS)

There are many studies underway, funded by foundations, government, and industry, to create an artificial pancreas. Such a device would function like an "autopilot" or "thermostat" which continuously measures glucose levels and would direct the timely release of insulin into the body. Currently available continuous glucose monitoring devices and insulin pumps function in an open-loop manner, requiring input from the parent/family. The artificial pancreas system would be a "closed loop" system — in other words it would work automatically, just like a pancreas.

SmartInsulin

SmartInsulin is an insulin that will make it possible to maintain a normal blood glucose level. The goal is to prevent both high and low blood glucose levels. It is in pre-clinical trials (not in people yet) but one hopes that it will be available in the future.

Research

Clinical Research

Nationwide there are over 450 clinical research studies being conducted in the area of type 1 diabetes. The ClinicalTrials.gov web site lists the titles of a wide array of type 1 diabetes research topics — from continuous glucose monitoring to Skittles, including:

- Randomized Trial to Assess Efficacy and Safety of Continuous Glucose Monitoring in Children 4-<8 Years With T1DM
- School Centered Telemedicine Program for Children with Type 1 Diabetes Mellitus
- Lantus in the Treatment of Type 1 Diabetes Children
- Skittles Effective for Treating Hypoglycemia in Children with Type 1 Diabetes
- The Protégé Study - Clinical Trial of MGA031 in Children and Adults with Recent Onset Type 1 Diabetes Mellitus
- Prospective Study of the Impact of Insulin Pump Therapy in Young Children with Type 1 Diabetes

Joslin Pediatrics Studies

We at Joslin are a big part of the research effort. The Joslin Pediatric Research team, along with the Joslin Clinic team, has a multitude of ongoing clinical research studies. Your child and/or your family may be eligible for participation in a trial. It is part of our mission to work towards better care for people with diabetes through research. We have the resources — experienced and knowledgeable Principal Investigators and staff, a Committee on Human Studies, as well as willing and able study participants — you!

The Pediatric, Adolescent, and Young Adult Section at Joslin is always involved in research. We continue to study:

- Technologies
- Continuous glucose monitoring
- Insulin pump therapy
- Causes of type 1 diabetes
- Genetics of diabetes
- Immunology of type 1 diabetes
- Pediatric type 2 diabetes
- Nutrition support for diabetes management
- Family teamwork in type 1 diabetes treatment

Joslin's Research Team

Joslin's Research Team represents the most comprehensive and dynamic research program anywhere in the world dedicated exclusively to diabetes. Nowhere else under one roof can you find such a breadth of diabetes research knowledge and treatment expertise. More than 300 scientists at Joslin are committed to pursuing innovative pathways of discovery to prevent, treat and cure type 1 and type 2 diabetes and their complications. Some of the most important historical discoveries and improvements in diabetes care worldwide were developed at Joslin.

Summary

Over the last 10 years, the diabetes community has benefited from the development and refinement of:

- Smarter glucose meters and insulin pumps
- Real-time continuous BG monitoring technology
- Point of care A1C testing
- 5 new insulins
- Electronic communications
- Genetic screening

These technological advances offer people with diabetes, their families, and healthcare providers new approaches to managing pediatric type1 diabetes with improved glycemic control and quality of life. What may the future look like in terms of diabetes management? A closed loop or artificial pancreas will bring more technologic advances and approach a cure for type 1 diabetes to improve the lives of all children, teens and adults with diabetes.

References and Resources

Strowig SM, Raskin P. Improved glycemic control in intensively treated type 1 diabetic patients using blood glucose meters with storage capability and computer-assisted analyses. *Diabetes Care*. 1998;21(10):1694-1698.

Laffel LMB, Hsu WC, McGill JB, Meneghini L, Volkening LK on behalf of the Monitoring of Blood Glucose Study Group. Continued use of an integrated meter with electronic logbook maintains improvements in glycemic control beyond a randomized, controlled trial. *Diabetes Technol Ther*. 2007;9(3);254-264.

Hirsch IB. Blood glucose monitoring technology: translating data into practice. *Endocr Pract*. 2004;10:67-76.

Hanauer D, Wentzell K, Laffel N, Laffel LMB. Computerized automated reminder diabetes system (CARDS): Web and SMS cell phone text messaging reminders to support diabetes management. ADA 2005.

Kumar VS, Wentzell KJ, Mikkelsen T, Pentland A, Laffel LM. The DAILY (Daily Automated Intensive Log for Youth) trial: a wireless, portable system to improve adherence and glycemic control in youth with diabetes. *Diabetes Technol Ther*. 2004;6(4):445-453.

Heidgerken AD, Adkins J, Storch EA, Williams L, Lewin AB, Silverstein JH, Malasanos T, Geffken GR. Telehealth intervention for adolescents with type 1 diabetes. *J Pediatr*. 2006;148(5):707-708.

Web site:

- National Institutes of Health. Clinical Trials. Clinical Trials Website: www.clinicaltrials.gov

19

The Top 10 Lessons Learned from Joslin Families

We hope you have enjoyed reading *Joslin's Guide to Managing Childhood Diabetes – A Family Teamwork Approach* as much as we enjoyed putting it together. We also hope that you will use this book as a reference tool in the days, weeks, and months ahead.

While we learn the most from our own experiences, we are sometimes fortunate to learn from the experiences of others. This final chapter takes the opportunity to list the top ten lessons learned from Joslin families in the day-to-day management of childhood diabetes.

Diabetes is a human condition. As humans, we must accept that we take false steps from time to time. Thus, if one or more of these pitfalls befalls you and your family, take solace in the recognition that many families have experienced these common mishaps before you. While the lessons learned are listed 1-10, they are equally common and equally challenging. Place no emphasis on the order in which they appear.

1. **Switching Insulin Doses** Insulin dosing for those treated by injection therapy varies by time of day, meal content, and blood glucose level. The morning dose is usually larger than the evening dose. By accident, it is quite easy to give the morning dose at night, which results in more insulin being administered than is normally prescribed. If this error occurs, do not panic. Call your healthcare team and discuss approaches to management; but mainly realize that you will view the evening now as morning and proceed with the expected food intake that would follow a morning dose of insulin. Frequent blood glucose monitoring will also be necessary.
2. **Switching Insulin Types** Insulin comes in multiple types with rapid-, short-, intermediate-, and long-acting varieties. Occasionally, it

is possible to get things confused and mistakenly give the rapid-acting insulin in place of the long-acting insulin or vice versa. If the wrong type of insulin is accidentally administered, call your child's healthcare team for advice. If too much rapid-acting insulin is given, your child will likely need to eat significantly more carbohydrates. In rare instances, rescue with a glucagon injection or possibly IV fluids might be needed.

3. **Missing Insulin Doses** Everyone gets tired at the end of a long day. Therefore, it is not unusual for a bedtime dose of insulin to be accidentally missed. Likewise, it is not unusual to forget to reconnect your child's insulin pump after an evening shower or bath. It is important to have a system of checks and balances in place to reduce the chances of these errors occurring. A double-check that an insulin pump has been reconnected after a shower or a bath goes a long way to ensuring consistent overnight insulin delivery. If you have forgotten either to give your child an insulin injection or to reconnect your child's pump prior to bedtime, it is important to check your child's blood glucose and ketone levels as soon as the error is detected so that an appropriate dose of insulin can be administered. Call your healthcare team for guidance if you are unsure of the proper dose.
4. **Withholding Insulin during Illness** Illnesses are common in growing children. A very common childhood illness is a stomach flu with nausea and vomiting. Since insulin is always given to cover the carbohydrates in food, a very common misconception is to withhold insulin when the appetite is diminished. Even in the setting of a stomach flu with decreased appetite and vomiting, your child needs insulin. The dose may need to be decreased but insulin must always be given. How much insulin to give is based upon the blood glucose and ketone levels, as well as your child's appetite. As discussed in Chapter 11: Sick Days and DKA Prevention, if your child is sick and vomiting, never withhold insulin and call your healthcare team for guidance.
5. **Continuing to Bolus via the Insulin Pump despite Multiple High Blood Glucose Levels** Insulin pumps are excellent tools that can be used to assist in the management of your child's diabetes. And although they

look quite smart, pumps present their own unique challenges. It is not uncommon for the insulin delivery catheter to kink without the pump alarming. As a result of inadequate insulin delivery, your child's blood glucose level may rise. A common error with a rising blood glucose level is for the family to continue to try to bolus insulin via the pump. Pump guidelines remind us all that two blood glucose values above 250 mg/dL should prompt us to do the following: first, check for ketones; second, give insulin via a syringe rather than the pump; third, change the entire pump setup. More times than not, upon changing the pump setup, the family sees a kinked catheter. Another pump pitfall, though uncommon, involves the inadvertent administration of long-acting basal insulin (*e.g.*, glargine, detemir) by the pump rather than a rapid-acting insulin (*e.g.*, lispro, aspart, glulisine). Insulin pumps are only to be used with rapid-acting insulin. If you find elevated blood glucose levels while using your child's pump, remember that his or her diabetes healthcare team is just a phone call away.

6. **Using Only Rapid-Acting Insulin** In the current era of mail-order pharmacies, many families receive insulin via the mail as a 3-month supply. Despite planning, however, it is possible to run out of insulin prior to receiving the delivery. We have heard of families who have run out of intermediate- or long-acting insulin and have resorted to administering only the rapid-acting insulin twice daily. This practice results in extremely high blood glucose values because there is no intermediate- (NPH) or long-acting insulin (glargine or detemir) on board. Therefore, if you find yourself without the appropriate insulin while awaiting a delivery, always contact a member of your child's healthcare team who will be able to assist you.
7. **Giving the Same Injection Twice or Improperly Mixed Insulin** We have already talked about what to do if your child's insulin dose is missed or delayed. Now we should also talk about what to do if your child's insulin dose is given twice or mixed improperly. Many families have both parents sharing in the care of the child with diabetes. With nothing but the best of intentions, one parent may administer an insulin dose and the second parent may administer

the dose again, not realizing that it had already been given. If twice as much insulin has been given, it is likely that twice as much food will need to be eaten. Remember to call your healthcare team for guidance in problem solving this dilemma. It is also possible to accidentally mix insulin in the wrong manner. For example, if intermediate-acting insulin (NPH) is drawn into a syringe before rapid-acting insulin, it is likely that the intermediate-acting insulin will contaminate the rapid-acting insulin bottle and alter the rapid-acting insulin's usual and expected mode of action. If this occurs, your healthcare team may advise you to discard the contaminated vial of insulin.

8. **Taking Rapid-Acting Insulin without Eating** Often, families are so busy during the week they long for weekend days with the opportunity to sleep a little late. In an effort to maintain a schedule of insulin administration, a child or teen may receive his or her morning insulin injection early on a weekend morning and then fall back asleep. It can be risky to go back to sleep after taking morning insulin without eating breakfast. This common pitfall can result in a significant low blood glucose level while your child is asleep. With your healthcare providers, discuss the best ways to increase flexibility around the timing of insulin administration so that your family can get a good night's rest on weekends and holidays.
9. **Forgetting to Synchronize Clocks on Diabetes Equipment** It is not unusual for children and families to use multiple blood glucose meters. This practice requires careful synchronization of the clocks on all the meters and especially on the insulin pump so that the downloaded data can reveal a consistent picture of blood glucose levels and insulin delivery. Incorrect time setting can be a particular challenge when families travel across time zones and forget to change the time on an insulin pump. This practice can result in daytime basal insulin rates being delivered overnight with resulting wide swings in blood glucose levels. Periodically check the times on all of your child's meters and/or insulin pump, especially in the spring and fall with daylight savings time and the return to standard time.
10. **Mis-Matching Syringe Lengths or Insulin Types in Insulin Infusers** Finally, one may use a new tool to help with insulin delivery by injec-

tion. Some of these new tools include a device called an Inject-ease or button-infuser such as the I-Port or Insulfon. Although these devices can aid in simplifying insulin delivery, they can also result in problems. For example, the Inject-ease requires the use of an adapter that matches the size of the insulin syringe being used by the child. If too large an adapter is used, the insulin syringe needle will not penetrate the skin enough to adequately deliver insulin. With use of button-infusers, it is important to avoid using the same infusion set for both rapid- and long-acting insulin due to altered insulin action through the button-infuser. Therefore, if you have any concerns, be sure to address them with your child's healthcare team.

While this list is not exhaustive, it gives you a flavor of the myriad of missteps that can occur in the management of diabetes. Most of these are tiny missteps and make absolutely no difference in the big picture of the life of your child. On the rare occasion that one of these missteps results in a severe low blood glucose level or a severe high glucose level with ketones, call your healthcare team and/or seek help from a local emergency room.

Conclusion

We live in an era where wonderful new approaches to diabetes management provide opportunities to maintain normal growth and development prevent complications preserve the health and protect the futures of children living with diabetes. By working together with your child's healthcare team, you can take advantage of these wonderful opportunities and be aware that when challenges arise there is help to get past them all. Just remember, it takes a village to raise a child and it takes a team to care for a child with diabetes.

Glossary

A1C – A blood test that measures average blood glucose over the past 2-3 months and is the best way to measure overall glucose control. It should be measured 2-4 times a year and the goal is less than 8.5% for children between the ages of 0 to 6 years old, less than 8% for children between the ages of 6 to 12 years old and less than 7.5% in teenagers between the ages of 13 to 19 years old.

Acanthosis nigricans – A thickening and darkening of the skin in patchy areas in the skin folds of the armpits, neck or groin, the color ranging from tan to dark brown. This is usually a sign of insulin resistance.

Aerobic exercise – Exercise in which the work performed by the muscles use oxygen when deriving energy from glucose. Aerobic means "with oxygen."

Alternative site glucose monitoring – Refers to the glucose level obtained with the use of a lancet device at an alternative site (other than fingertip) such as the forearm or base of the thumb. Glucose levels from alternative sites may occasionally differ from plasma glucose levels from fingersticks because of the lag effect (see Lag effect below). This lag effect is also noted with interstitial glucose measurements compared to plasma glucose measurements.

Anaerobic exercise – Exercise in which the work performed by the muscles does not use oxygen when deriving energy from glucose. Anaerobic means "without oxygen."

Antibodies – Proteins that the body makes to protect itself from foreign substances such as bacteria and viruses.

Autoantibodies – Proteins the immune system produces which act against the body's own cells. Some are destructive and can cause symptoms or a disease, while others may only be a marker of a disease such as type 1 diabetes.

Autoimmune disease – Disorder of the body's immune system in which the immune system mistakenly attacks and destroys body tissue considered foreign.

Basal insulin – The insulin that controls blood glucose levels between meals and overnight. It controls glucose in the fasting state. The basal insulin is provided as the basal rate by a pump or as the long-acting insulin injected by syringe or pen. Basal insulin is approximately half of the total daily insulin dose.

Basal/bolus therapy – Refers to a specific kind of physiologic insulin replacement in which basal insulin is provided with a long-acting insulin analog and bolus insulin is provided with a rapid-acting insulin analog aimed at covering elevated blood glucoses and the carbohydrates contained in meals and snacks. Treatment via an insulin pump may also be referred to in this way.

Beta cells – Cells that produce insulin. They are located within the islets of Langerhans in the pancreas.

Blood glucose (or just glucose or blood sugar) – A type of sugar that is created when the carbohydrate that one eats is broken down in the body. During digestion, glucose passes through the wall of the intestine into the bloodstream to the liver and eventually into the general circulation. From there, glucose can then enter individual cells or tissues throughout the body to be used for fuel and provide energy.

Blood pressure – The pressure against the walls of your blood vessels. High blood pressure is more common in persons with diabetes.

Body mass index (BMI) – A method of determining by the relationship between height and weight whether or not a person is obese, overweight, underweight, or of normal weight.

Bolus – A dose of insulin given in addition to the basal insulin to either correct a high blood glucose and/or cover carbs at a meal or snack.

Bolus insulin – A burst of insulin that is delivered by injection or by the insulin pump to cover a meal or snack or to correct for a high blood glucose level.

Calibration – Term that refers to setting the new glucose sensor technology to accurately measure interstitial glucose levels. Calibration occurs by checking a fingerstick blood glucose level and entering that glucose level into the continuous glucose monitor.

Carbohydrate (Carb) – The main source of fuel for the body. Carbohydrates include starches and sugars and are found in bread, pasta, fruits, vegetables, milk, and sweets. Carbs are broken down into a sugar called glucose.

Carbohydrate counting – A meal planning method commonly used by people with diabetes to plan their food and meal choices. Carbohydrate counting helps one achieve a balance between the amount of carbohydrate foods eaten and the available insulin.

Celiac Disease – An autoimmune disease that affects 6-14% of individuals with type 1 diabetes. Treatment is the removal of all gluten-containing grains (wheat, barley, and rye) from the meal plan.

Charcot Foot – A condition in which the small bones of the foot become misaligned, leading to foot deformity. It is a problem that can evolve as a result of nerve damage.

Child Life Specialists – Pediatric professionals who work with patients, families, and others involved in the child's care in order to help them manage stress and their understanding in a medical setting.

Cholesterol – A fat-like substance that is manufactured in the liver or intestines, but is also found in some of the foods we eat. (Only animal foods, such as eggs, milk, cheese, liver, meat, and poultry contain cholesterol.)

Chronological age – The number of years an individual has lived.

Cognitive behavioral therapy (CBT) – A therapeutic approach that examines a person's thinking patterns to help the patient redirect negative thinking patterns into more positive thinking patterns, because it is believed that a person's thinking patterns influences one's behavior.

Continuous Glucose Monitoring (CGM) Technology – A device that continuously measures the glucose level in the body fluid surrounding the cells in the interstitial fluid. There are several different devices, which work in similar ways. Each requires the placement of a small electrode — called the sensor — just under the skin in the fatty tissue. A transmitter is placed on the skin on top of the sensor. The transmitter sends the glucose data wirelessly to a receiver. The receiver provides the glucose readings every 1-5 minutes, depending on the particular device. These glucose readings do not replace fingerstick blood glucose monitoring but can provide important trends for rising or falling blood glucoses as well as alarms when the glucose level is out of range. The sensor is inserted much like a pump infusion set and needs to be calibrated and changed every 3-7 days according to the manufactures' policies.

Consolidated Omnibus Budget Reconciliation Act (COBRA) – A temporary continuation of health insurance coverage.

CSII – Continuous subcutaneous insulin infusion, otherwise know as pump therapy.

Correction factor (CF) – A term used for the insulin dosage required to lower blood glucose to a specified target level. Correction levels are often used for patients receiving insulin pump therapy or basal/bolus multiple injection therapy. A correction factor of 1 to 50 means 1 unit of insulin will drop a blood glucose 50 points. The correction factor is also called the sensitivity factor (SF). Correction factors usually vary person-to-person and even throughout the day.

Dawn phenomenon – A rise in blood glucose levels that occurs in the early morning hours due to changing hormone levels.

Dehydration – Excessive loss of body water.

Diabetes educator – A healthcare worker who has the skill and knowledge to teach a person with diabetes how to manage the condition. Diabetes educators may be doctors, nurses, dietitians, mental health, or fitness clinicians. Some also have the credential CDE (Certified Diabetes Educator).

Diabetic ketoacidosis (also called ketoacidosis or DKA) – A condition that results from a lack of sufficient insulin in the body, leading to high blood glucose levels and ketone formation. It is an extremely serious and life-threatening condition that may lead to coma and death. The symptoms of ketoacidosis are nausea, stomach pain, vomiting, chest pain, rapid shallow breathing and difficulty staying awake.

Diabetes Mellitus – A chronic medical condition characterized by elevated levels of glucose (sugar) in the blood. Diabetes requires life-long therapy.

Dietitian or Registered Dietitian (RD) – A healthcare provider who specializes in food, nutrition and meal planning.

Disordered eating – A less severe eating disturbance that does not meet the criteria for anorexia nervosa or bulimia nervosa.

eAG (estimated Average Glucose) – A new way to present an A1C value in numbers like you see on your child's blood glucose meter. Average glucose = (28.7 x A1C) – 46.7.

Eating disorder – A severe eating disturbance that meets the criteria for anorexia nervosa or bulimia nervosa.

EMLA cream – A topical anesthetic that numbs the skin and decreases the sensation of pain.

Endocrinologist – A doctor who specializes in diseases of the endocrine system, such as diabetes.

Exercise lag effect – A term that refers to the hypoglycemia (low blood glucose) that may occur anywhere from 1-2 hours after exercise to as many as 8-10 hours after exercise. The exercise lag effect results from the muscles in the body replenishing their stored glucose by extracting glucose from the blood stream.

Exercise Physiologist – A healthcare provider that specializes in how the human body functions during physical activity.

Fasting blood glucose test – A blood test in which a sample of blood is drawn after an overnight fast to measure the amount of glucose in the blood.

Fingerstick – The method by which blood glucose is checked by obtaining a small drop of blood using a lancet at the tip of the finger.

Gastroenterologist – A doctor who specializes in the condition and diseases of the gastrointestinal (GI) tract.

Glucagon – A hormone normally produced by the pancreas that is released when the blood glucose is low, causing the liver to release stored glucose (glycogen) into the bloodstream.

Glucose – A simple form of sugar that is created when the body's digestive processes break down the food we eat. Glucose is the body's main source of energy.

Glucose meter – A device that measures one's blood glucose levels.

Glucose tolerance test (GTT) – A test used to diagnose diabetes. Blood tests are done every hour or at the 2-hour point after drinking a sugar-filled liquid. If at 2 hours, the blood glucose rises to over 200 mg/dL, diabetes is diagnosed. This test is not as common as a fasting glucose test.

Glycogen – Glucose that is stored in muscles and liver.

Glycemic Index (GI) – A system of ranking foods containing equal amounts of carbohydrate according to how much they raise blood glucose levels. For instance, the carbohydrate in a slice of 100% stone-ground whole wheat bread (a low glycemic index food) may have less impact on blood glucose than a slice of processed white bread (a high glycemic index food). The GI is an additional meal-planning tool to help one understand how carbohydrate foods can differ in their effects on blood glucose.

Glycemic load (GL) – A system of ranking carbohydrate foods based on how much they raise blood glucose levels that combines the GI value and the carbohydrate content of an average serving of a food, of a meal, or of a day's worth of food.

HDL (high-density lipoprotein — also called "good" cholesterol) – A type of blood cholesterol that sweeps excess cholesterol from the blood back to the liver where it is reprocessed or eliminated.

Hemoglobin A1C – The measure of average blood glucose levels over the previous 2-3 months. Hemoglobin A1C is often referred to as a blood glucose with a memory.

Honeymoon – Once a child starts on insulin shots, the remaining beta cells get a rest and allow the pancreas to produce some insulin for a time.

Hormones – Chemical messengers made in one part of the body to transfer "information" through the bloodstream to cells in another part of the body. Insulin is a hormone.

Hyperglycemia – High blood glucose levels. Blood glucose is generally considered high when it is 180 mg/dL or greater or above your individual blood glucose target.

Hyperosmolar hyperglycemic state (HHS) – A serious condition resulting from extremely high levels of blood glucose, causing excessive urination and severe dehydration, but without ketones. It is not very common.

Hypertension – High blood pressure (blood flows through the blood vessels with a greater than normal force), which is defined as blood pressure equal to or greater than norm for a child's age and height.

Hypoglycemia – Refers to low blood glucose levels below 80 mg/dL with or without symptoms or below 90 mg/dL with symptoms. Hypoglycemia usually results in symptoms such as shakiness, sweating, rapid heartbeat, hunger, headache, and trouble concentrating. Symptoms of hypoglycemia may vary person to person.

Hypoglycemia unawareness – A condition in which one does not recognizes the symptoms of low blood glucose.

Immunosuppression – Involves an act that reduces the effectiveness and efficiency of the immune system.

Impaired fasting glucose (IFG) – A fasting glucose level between 100 mg/dL and 125 mg/dL. Fasting blood test results between these numbers mean that you have pre-diabetes.

Impaired glucose tolerance (IGT) – A blood glucose level after a 2-hour glucose tolerance test between 140 and 199 mg/dL. A test result between these numbers means you have pre-diabetes or are at risk for diabetes.

Infusion set – Plastic tubing used with an insulin pump.

Insulin – A hormone made in the pancreas that helps glucose pass into the cells where it is used to create energy for the body.

Insulin pen – An insulin delivery method that looks like a writing pen.

Insulin pump – A small, battery powered insulin delivery system; a mechanical device, typically the size of a beeper or small cell phone that releases insulin into the tissues of the body by way of tubing and a needle.

Insulin reaction (hypoglycemia) – Low blood glucose resulting from too much insulin, too much activity or too little food.

Insulin resistance – A condition that makes it harder for the cells to properly use insulin.

Insulin sensitivity factor (also called the correction factor) – The amount of blood glucose measured in mg/dL that is lowered by 1 unit of rapid-acting or regular insulin. The insulin sensitivity factor is used to calculate the amount of insulin needed to return blood glucose to within your target blood glucose range.

Insulin-to-Carbohydrate Ratio (I:Carb) – A method of determining how much rapid-acting insulin is needed to cover the carbohydrate eaten at a meal or snack. This is used as part of a more advanced level of carbohydrate counting.

Intensification – Insulin-producing beta cell destruction continues. The child's blood glucoses continue to get more difficult to stay in range.

Intermediate-acting insulin – A type of insulin that begins to work to lower blood glucose within 1-4 hours and works hardest 4-15 hours after injection. The intermediate-acting insulin is NPH.

Interstitial glucose – Refers to the glucose level measured with the use of continuous glucose sensing technology. The institium or interstitial space refers to the area between the body's cells bathed by body fluids.

Islet cells – Cells in the pancreas that make insulin (beta cells) or glucagon (alpha cells).

Ketones – Acids produced due to lack of enough insulin to use the glucose in the bloodstream for energy. The body turns to its fat stores for energy when there is insufficient insulin. When this occurs, ketones are produced, which accumulate in the blood and spill into the urine. These ketones are made when fat is metabolized as a source of energy. The excessive formation of ketones in the blood is called *ketosis*, and the presence of ketones in the urine is called *ketonuria*. Allowed to go untreated, the combination of high blood glucose and ketones can lead to *ketoacidosis* (also called DKA).

Ketonuria – The presence of ketones in the urine.

Ketosis – The excessive formation of ketones in the blood.

Lactose Intolerance – The inability to digest lactose, the sugar found in milk.

Lag effect – Refers to the delay in the rise or fall of a glucose level measured either in the interstitial space or at alternative sites when compared to fingerstick blood glucose monitoring.

Lancet – A small needle used to get a drop of blood from the finger, arm, or other site. The blood is placed on a special strip, which is put into the blood glucose meter. The meter reads the strip and gives a blood glucose reading.

Lancing device – The piece of equipment that holds the lancet. It has a spring-like mechanism that releases the needle towards the fingertip.

Lifestyle changes – Changes made to one's eating habits and physical activity in order to control blood glucose.

Long-acting peakless – A type of basal insulin that begins to work to lower blood glucose within 1-2 hours after injection and works for 24 hours. The long-acting peakless insulins are glargine and detemir.

LDL (low-density lipoprotein) – A type of blood cholesterol that is considered "bad" because it can be deposited in the arteries, increasing the risk of heart attack or stroke.

Maturity Onset Diabetes of the Young (MODY) – An inherited genetic disorder of beta cells. In this condition, the beta cell is not destroyed, but it is unable to function properly to make or release insulin.

Medical Assistant – A person trained to assist medical professionals.

Medical Nutrition Therapy (MNT) – A method of controlling blood glucose by working with a dietitian to assess one's food and nutrition needs and then developing and following an individualized meal plan.

Metabolism – The process by which the cells of the body change food so that it can be used for energy or so that it can be used to build or maintain cells and tissues.

Metabolic syndrome – A cluster of conditions that increase the risk of developing vascular disease (heart disease, strokes, and peripheral vascular disease). The most recognizable components of this syndrome are abdominal obesity, high blood pressure (hypertension), high triglycerides (part of the lipid profile), low HDL (the "good" cholesterol), and glucose intolerance.

Microalbumin test – A urine test that measures the presence of small amounts of a protein called albumin.

Microalbuminuria – The presence of small amounts of albumin, a protein, in the urine.

Milligram per deciliter (mg/dL) – The standard measure of blood glucose in the United States.

Millimolar (mMol) – The standard measure of blood glucose in other countries. Glucose in millimoles multiplied by 18 provides the glucose level in milligram per deciliter.

Mixed dose – An injection that contains two or more types of insulin given in the same syringe at the same time.

Multiple daily injections – A form of insulin therapy in which blood glucose levels are controlled and carbohydrates in the meal plan are managed through the delivery of insulin given through multiple injections.

Nephrologis – A doctor who specializes in conditions of the kidney.

Neurologist – A doctor who specializes in conditions of the nervous system.

Nocturnal hypoglycemia – Low blood glucose that occurs in the middle of the night.

Noncaloric or non-nutritive sweeteners – Sweeteners that contribute few, if any, calories and have no affect on blood glucose levels.

Nonproliferative retinopathy – The initial stage in diabetic retinopathy. High levels of blood glucose cause damage to the blood vessels in the retina. The blood vessels leak fluid, which can collect and cause the retina to swell.

Nutritive or caloric sweeteners – Sweeteners that contribute calories and can affect blood glucose levels.

Ophthalmologist – A doctor specializing in conditions and surgeries of the eyes.

Optometrist (OD) – A healthcare provider who is trained and licensed to provide eye care.

Oral glucose-lowering medications (also referred to as oral antidiabetes medications) – "Diabetes pills," which are used in combination with a meal plan and physical activity, as well as in combination with each other, and sometimes with insulin to control blood glucose levels.

Pancreas – An organ located in the abdomen with two functions: some cells provide enzymes to assist in digestion and the specialized beta cells that are part of the endocrine system and produce the hormone insulin. These insulin-producing cells are located in the tail of the pancreas in an area called the islets.

Pathophysiology – Changes that occur within an organ or tissue due to disease.

Physiologic insulin therapy (also called intensive insulin therapy) – An insulin program that attempts to provide insulin in the way that your body would if you didn't have diabetes. Insulin is adjusted to accommodate your food intake and your activity level, and as a result insulin doses change from one day to the next.

Plasma glucose – The glucose level measured with the aid of a fingerstick.

Polycystic ovary syndrome (PCOS) – A hormone imbalance that can cause irregular periods, unwanted hair growth, and acne in teens and young women.

Pre-diabetes – A condition in which either the fasting or 2-hour post-meal blood glucose levels are higher than normal, but not high enough for a diagnosis of type 2 diabetes. Studies show that most people with pre-diabetes will develop type 2 diabetes within 10 years if they don't change their lifestyle. They also have a higher risk of developing cardiovascular disease.

Proliferative retinopathy – A more serious stage of diabetic retinopathy in which there is a greater loss of vision or even total blindness. During this stage, abnormal blood vessels grow over the surface of the retina.

Protein – One of the main nutrients from food along with carbohydrate and fat. The body uses protein to build and repair body tissue. Muscles, organs, bones, skin, and many of the hormones in the body are made from protein. As a secondary role, protein can also provide energy for the body if carbohydrate is not available. Food sources of protein include meat, poultry, fish, eggs, dairy products, and beans.

Psychologist – A mental-health professional.

Rapid-acting insulin – A type of insulin that begins to work to lower blood glucose within 10-30 minutes and works hardest 30 minutes to 3 hours after injection. There are 3 approved rapid-acting insulins: lispro, aspart, and glulisine.

Rebound hyperglycemia (high blood glucose or the Somogyi phenomenon) – A condition in which, because blood glucose levels are too low, the counter-regulatory or stress hormones cause the liver to release too much glucose.

Receiver – The component of continuous glucose monitoring technology which displays the interstitial glucose with values in numeric and graphical forms. Some transmitters provide arrows to indicate trending information.

Retina – The thin, light-sensitive inner lining in the back of your eye.

Retinopathy – Damage to the *retina*, the thin, light-sensitive inner lining in the back of the eye. This damage occurs to small blood vessels in the retina which are easily harmed by high levels of glucose in the blood.

Saline – Sterile salt water.

Saturated fat – A type of food fat that is solid at room temperature. Saturated fats raise blood cholesterol levels by interfering with the entry of cholesterol into cells, causing cholesterol to remain in the bloodstream longer and to become a part of the plaque that builds up in the blood vessels.

Self-monitoring – Managing one's diabetes by checking blood glucose, being aware of food intake, physical activity, and medication, and being aware of how each of these elements work together in order to keep blood glucose in control.

SMBG (self-monitoring of blood glucose) – Checking your blood glucose with a blood glucose meter.

Sensitivity Factor (also called the correction factor) – The number of points (mg/dL) the blood glucose will drop after 1 unit of insulin is given

Sensor – The part of the continuous glucose monitoring technology with a filament, or probe, that sits under the skin in the interstitial space and is taped onto the skin. Once inserted, this sensor remains in place, virtually painlessly, for 3-7 days, according to manufacturer guidelines.

Sensor noise – Refers to the signal occasionally picked up by a continuous glucose sensor that interferes with the interstitial glucose measurement and leads to some temporary loss of sensor accuracy.

Sensor warm up – Refers to the period of time in which a glucose sensor is calibrating in order to measure accurate glucose levels. The sensor warm up varies according to the sensor technology, anywhere from 2-10 hours.

Short-acting insulin – A type of insulin that begins to work to lower blood glucose within 30-60 minutes and works hardest 1-5 hours after injection. The common form of short-acting insulin is called *regular*.

Single dose – An injection that contains one type of insulin.

Sugar alcohols or polyols – Sweeteners that replace other sugars in foods, causing slightly lower rises in blood glucose.

Target blood glucose or target glucose – Reflects the goal glucose value used to calculate the insulin dosage needed to correct (or lower) an elevated glucose value. The target number is used in calculating the insulin dosage with the insulin-to-carb ratio. There are positive corrections in which elevated blood glucoses are corrected down to a target number. There are also negative corrections in which low blood glucoses are corrected up to a target number. With positive corrections, insulin is given. With negative corrections, insulin is usually taken away from a dose that would be provided with a meal or snack. Generally, people have a target range and aim to keep the majority (over 50%) of glucose levels within that range, often 70 to 150 mg/dL. The target range varies person to person.

Transmitter – The part of the continuous glucose sensing technology which sits upon the glucose sensor and wirelessly transmits data to the separate receiver.

Trans fats – A type of fat formed from *hydrogenation*, a chemical process that changes a liquid oil into a solid fat. Trans fats are found in processed foods, such as snack foods, cookies, fast foods, and some stick or solid margarines. They can raise cholesterol levels and should be eaten in as small amounts as possible.

Trend – A glucose trend reflects either a rise or fall of blood glucose levels. Glucose trends are evident with the use of continuous glucose sensor technology.

Trend correction – A new term that designates the change in insulin dosage depending upon whether the glucose level is rising or falling, as revealed with continuous glucose sensing technology. Trend corrections usually vary from 10-20% whether the glucose level is changing 30-60 mg/dL per hour or greater than 60 mg/dL per hour, respectively. Some sensors provide trend data with up or down arrows or up or down double arrows.

Triglycerides – A type of fat stored in fat cells as body fat and burned for energy. High levels of triglycerides are linked with an increased risk of heart and blood vessel disease.

Total Daily Dose (TDD) – The total number of units of all insulins used in a 24 hour period.

Unsaturated fat (both *polyunsaturated* and *monounsaturated*) – Fats that come primarily from vegetables and are liquid at room temperature. Polyunsaturated fats can help lower cholesterol levels. Monounsaturated fats also help lower blood cholesterol levels and may help to raise HDL cholesterol levels.

Index